Patient Safety in Anatomic and Clinical Pathology Laboratories

Deborah Sesok-Pizzini, MD, MBA
Editor

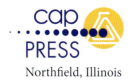

Northfield, Illinois

Copyright © 2017 College of American Pathologists (CAP).
All rights reserved. None of the contents of this publication may be reproduced, stored in a retrieval system, or transmitted in any form or by any means (electronic, mechanical, photocopying, recording, or otherwise) without prior written permission of the publisher.

The inclusion of a vendor, company, product name, or service in a CAP publication should not be construed as an endorsement of such vendor, company, product, or service, nor is failure to include the name of a vendor, company, product, or service to be construed as disapproval.

Library of Congress Control Number: 2017932182
ISBN: 978-194109636-9

Printed in the USA

College of American Pathologists
325 Waukegan Road
Northfield, Illinois 60093
800-323-4040
cap.org

Contents

	Contributors	iv
	Preface	v
1	Introduction *Tina Ipe, MD, MPH; Lee Hilborne, MD, MPH, DLM(ASCP)*	1
2	The Culture of Patient Safety in the Laboratory *Frederick L. Kiechle, MD, PhD*	5
3	Human Factors and Patient Safety in the Laboratory *Scott R. Owens, MD*	19
4	Communication, Handoffs, and Transitions *Virginia Elizabeth Duncan, MD; Suzanne Renée Thibodeaux, MD, PhD; Gene P. Siegal, MD, PhD*	29
5	Utilizing Technology to Improve Laboratory Patient Safety *Anand S. Dighe, MD, PhD*	43
6	Tools and Methods to Improve and Evaluate Patient Safety in the Laboratory *Tina Ipe, MD, MPH; Lee Hilborne, MD, MPH*	61
7	Diagnostic Errors and Cognitive Bias *Stephen S. Raab, MD*	71
8	Building High-Reliability Teams in the Laboratory *Nicole D. Riddle, MD*	87
9	Developing a Patient Safety Curriculum for Resident and Fellow Education *Deborah Sesok-Pizzini, MD, MBA*	101
10	Patient Safety and the Patient Navigator *Elizabeth A. Wagar, MD*	111
	Index	119

Contributors

Deborah Sesok-Pizzini, MD, MBA
Chief, Blood Bank and Transfusion Medicine
Vice-Chief, Department of Pathology and Laboratory Medicine
Department Safety Officer, CHOP Pathology and Laboratory Medicine
Children's Hospital of Philadelphia
Professor of Clinical Pathology and Laboratory Medicine
Perelman School of Medicine at the University of Pennsylvania
Philadelphia, Pennsylvania

Anand S. Dighe, MD, PhD
Director, Massachusetts General Hospital Core Laboratory
Associate Professor, Harvard Medical School
Department of Pathology
Massachusetts General Hospital
Boston, Massachusetts

Virginia E. Duncan, MD
AP Chief Resident
Department of Pathology
University of Alabama at Birmingham
Birmingham, Alabama

Lee Hilborne, MD, MPH, DLM(ASCP)
Professor of Pathology and Laboratory Medicine
David Geffen School of Medicine at UCLA
Medical Director, Care Coordination, UCLA HealthSystem
Senior Medical Director, Medical Affairs
Quest Diagnostics, Inc.
Los Angeles, California

Tina Ipe, MD, MPH
Medical Director, Donor Services
Associate Medical Director, Transfusion Medicine
Assistant Professor of Pathology, Weill Cornell Medical College
Department of Pathology and Genomic Medicine
Houston Methodist Hospital
Houston, Texas

Frederick L. Kiechle, MD, PhD
Consultant
Clinical Pathology
Cooper City, Florida

Scott R. Owens, MD
Associate Professor of Pathology
Director, Division of Quality and Health Improvement
Medical Director of Professional Practice Evaluation
University of Michigan
Ann Arbor, Michigan

Stephen S. Raab, MD
University of Mississippi Medical Center
Jackson, Mississippi
Memorial University of Newfoundland and Labrador and Eastern Health
St. John's, Newfoundland

Nicole D. Riddle, MD
Pathologist and Laboratory Medical Director
Marshall Cancer Care Centers
Marshall County, Alabama
Cunningham Pathology
An Aurora Diagnostics Partner
Birmingham, Alabama

Gene P. Siegal, MD, PhD
RW Mowry Endowed Professor of Pathology
Executive Vice-Chair – Pathology, UAB Medicine
University of Alabama – Birmingham
Birmingham, Alabama

Suzanne Renée Thibodeaux, MD, PhD
Fellow, Blood Bank/Transfusion Medicine
Division of Transfusion Medicine and Therapeutic Pathology
Department of Pathology and Laboratory Medicine
Hospital of the University of Pennsylvania
Philadelphia, Pennsylvania

Elizabeth A. Wagar, MD
Professor and Chair, Department of Laboratory Medicine, Division of Pathology/Lab Medicine
Jose M. Trujillo Endowed Chair in Laboratory Medicine
The University of Texas MD Anderson Cancer Center
Houston, Texas

Preface

The patient safety movement in health care became energized after the publication of *To Err Is Human* by the Institute of Medicine in the 1990s. It was revealed how many medical errors occur in the health care system and how many were, in fact, preventable. Then, organizations such as the Joint Commission on Accreditation of Healthcare Organizations (JCAHO; now The Joint Commission) and the Accreditation Council for Graduate Medical Education (ACGME) began to regulate standards for implementation of patient safety into hospitals and training programs. In pathology in the early 1970s, regulations via the Clinical Laboratory Improvement Amendments (CLIA) required pathology laboratories to perform standardized testing with the necessity to show competency, proficiency, and reliability in patient care. In that sense, pathology was considered an early adopter and leader in patient safety along with another specialty, anesthesia.

Now, several years later, we continue to evolve in the area of patient safety with additional regulatory and reporting requirements from accrediting agencies that oversee hospitals, laboratories, and training programs. Hospital reporting of medical errors is now even required by many states so that these data can be analyzed to help preventable errors from occurring. Many institutions have committed to a major change when it comes to patient safety and have engaged in work groups such as the Institute for Healthcare Improvement (IHI) to help learn from one another and provide benchmarking data on achieving the goal of being a high-reliability organization.

In this book, we discuss patient safety in both the anatomic and clinical laboratories. We discuss the common types of errors we see in pathology, the human factors associated with these errors, and how communication and technology are important factors in reducing these errors. We also focus on tools and methods to improve patient safety and reduce the number of errors, and on how cognitive bias may play a role in contributing to these errors. Important aspects that will also be addressed are building high-reliability teams and the role of the patient navigator in helping to address some of the patient safety issues with regard to continuity, coordination, and care. Last, we will look at developing a patient safety curriculum in pathology and how the new accreditation milestones relate to advancing patient safety initiatives.

It is my pleasure to bring you this book, and I am grateful for the subject matter expert authors who contributed to this material. I am also thankful for the assistance of Caryn Tursky from the College of American Pathologists (CAP) for her editorial work on this book and to the CAP Publications Committee for having the vision to recognize the importance of this book for the practicing and in-training pathologist.

This book is dedicated to all of the current and future patients who will avoid preventable harm as a result of the influence of this book and other literature advancing patient safety.

1

Introduction

Tina Ipe, MD, MPH
Lee Hilborne, MD, MPH

Fifty years ago, Abraham Maslow stated that if you only have a hammer, you tend to see every problem as a nail. This analogy applies equally well to health care as to other aspects of life. Fortunately, over the last few decades, health care—and laboratory medicine in particular—have seen the emergence of numerous strategies and tools to improve patient safety and quality of care. In 1946, when Dr. William Sunderman developed the first proficiency testing service under the auspices of the American Society of Clinical Pathologists (ASCP; now American Society for Clinical Pathology), the predecessor to the College of American Pathologists (CAP) proficiency testing program that we know today, the laboratory had very limited tools to improve quality.[1,2] This chapter discusses the many tools that now exist in the laboratory professional's toolbox that can be applied to improve patient safety.

Any set of tools must be considered as a framework for strategies that can be brought to the table when solving problems. Depending on the specific scenario or scenarios involved, multiple approaches may be needed and specific tools adapted to effectively meet a particular challenge or question.

Current State of Patient Safety in the Laboratory

Medical errors are, for the most part, preventable; however, many patients experience significant morbidity and mortality as a result of medical errors in US hospitals. It is estimated that medical mistakes affect approximately 10% of hospitalized patients and cause hundreds of thousands of preventable deaths in hospitals each year.[3] When these adverse medical events are analyzed, the findings show that the system is faulty, rather than the personnel involved.[3] The adverse events stem from errors in prevention, diagnosis, and medication management.[4-6] Further breakdown of the diagnostic errors revealed that 50% were caused by failure to use indicated tests, 32% were due to inappropriate action based on test results, and 55% were the result of an avoidable delay in diagnosis.[5,6]

In September 2015, the Institute of Medicine (IOM) released an important report, *Improving Diagnosis in Health Care,*[7] which specifically acknowledged that diagnostic errors in health care have received very little attention even in the wake of the landmark IOM report published in 2000, *To Err Is Human.*[8] The 2015 report highlighted three specific themes:

- Diagnostic error has received relatively little attention in the last 15 years, in part because diagnostic error is underappreciated and data on diagnostic error is sparse.
- Partnering with patients and improving communication are critical to reduce diagnostic errors.
- Reducing diagnostic error requires teamwork and systems improvements, consistent with the messages from the initial IOM report.

Improving Diagnosis in Health Care calls on the medical profession—and the diagnostic medical communities in particular—to hone our tools and skills to better recognize, understand, and learn from diagnostic errors.

Patient safety initiatives involve a fair reporting and learning culture, where stakeholders understand the system and the processes that result in medical errors. From several studies, it is known that most medical errors occur outside the laboratory during the preanalytic and postanalytic phases. For the purposes of this chapter, the term *laboratory medicine* encompasses the medical subspecialties of molecular and genetic diagnostics, microbiology, transfusion medicine, clinical chemistry, anatomic pathology, and hematopathology. The analytic phase had the lowest frequency of errors (13.3%-15%).[9] In comparison, in the preanalytic and postanalytic phases, the frequency of errors occurred at 61.9% to 68.2% and 19.8% to 23.1%, respectively.[9] A recent cross-sectional study conducted at a teaching hospital showed similar high results for errors in the preanalytic phase of the total testing process at 65.1%, but postanalytic errors only occurred at 11.7%,[4] and analytic errors occurred at 23.2%, higher than previous publications on patient safety errors in the laboratory.[4]

In 2003, it was estimated that approximately 7 billion laboratory tests were performed annually in US laboratories.[6] Although laboratory medicine is only a small part of the hospital budget, it influences 60% to 70% of all critical decisions that affect downstream patient care.[10] Given this, patient safety can be affected adversely by laboratory processes such as sample misidentification, specimen quality, analytical quality, and laboratory results reporting. To date there have

Introduction

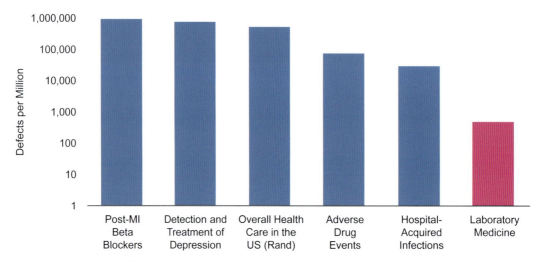

Figure 1-1. The laboratory has the lowest defects per million than the rest of health care (modified from Leape[3]). MI, myocardial infarction.

been many important studies that address patient safety in the laboratory. Some initiatives reviewed include more awareness of patient safety errors, institution of quality indicators and guidelines, and technological advances.[9] Among other challenges, ones that significantly impact laboratories and their processes are the following:
- Consolidation of hospital laboratories
- Delivery of services in a wide variety of settings
- Downsizing and shortage of laboratory personnel
- Decreased Medicare and other third-party payer reimbursements
- Alternative-site testing through options such as point-of-care testing
- Focus on test cost reduction and other financial incentives[10]

The understanding of the strengths and weaknesses of patient safety in the laboratory would not have occurred without important achievements that have brought patient safety to the forefront of health care. And now, with the publication of *Improving Diagnosis in Health Care*, we have been rechallenged to delve deeper into learning and implementing procedures that will enhance patient safety through improved laboratory processes and workflow.

The Evolution of Patient Safety Culture

During the early 1990s, the public developed a consciousness about patient safety. The Harvard Medical Practice Study I, published in 1991, was among the first studies to explore this topic and was the springboard for discussion in health care organizations.[11] The study's objective was to develop reliable estimates of the incidence of adverse events in hospitalized patients. The study showed that 3.7% of hospitalized patients suffered disabling injury caused by medical mismanagement rather than their underlying disease.[11] The study performed a retrospective review of 30,121 patient records from 51 nonfederal New York hospitals. It showed that in the 3.7% of adverse events, 70.5% resulted in less than 6 months of disability, 2.6% resulted in permanent disability, and 13.6% resulted in death.[11] Although the study first showcased the incidence of adverse events in hospitalized patients, public outcry and calls for change came with the publication of *To Err is Human: Building a Safer Health System* by the IOM in 2000.[8] The report noted that as many as 48,000 to 98,000 Americans died from adverse medical mistakes each year. In addition, the report asserted that the medical errors resulted from faulty systems rather than people, and proposed nonpunitive means to discover and ameliorate problems in health care system infrastructures. Subsequently, the IOM published *Crossing the Quality Chasm* in 2001.[12] This report highlighted that marginal reforms would inadequately address systemic flaws. The premise for changing systems is to improve patient safety by reducing loss of life and decreasing the overall economic burden caused by morbidity and mortality. And now *Improving Diagnosis in Health Care* confirms these findings. They state that 5% of US adults who seek outpatient care will experience diagnostic errors (inaccurate or delayed diagnosis), that diagnostic errors are the leading type of paid medical malpractice claims, and that most people will experience at least one diagnostic error during their lifetime, at times with devastating consequences.[7]

Patient safety improvement or quality improvement in health care was an emerging concept in the 1990s, but quality improvement as an approach to analyze performance and systems was conceptualized

Introduction

and actualized in the 1940s. It was initially used in the manufacturing industry by Joseph Duran and W. Edwards Deming to:
- Decrease production variation and error
- Increase reproducibility and reliability of the production process
- Improve production quality
- Decrease production cost[13]

In addition to manufacturing, health care organizations have utilized quality improvement tools from other industries, such as the aviation and nuclear power industries.

In the interim between the 1940s and 1990s, various health care agencies were established, such as The Joint Commission (originally the Joint Commission on Accreditation of Hospitals; 1951), IOM (1970), Accreditation Association for Ambulatory Health Care (AAAHC; 1979), the Agency for Healthcare Research and Quality (AHRQ; originally the Agency for Healthcare Policy and Research; 1989), and the Institute for Medical Quality (1995). In addition to the creation of various government, research, and accreditation agencies, Avedis Donabedian published his concept regarding how to effectively evaluate quality of medical care by dividing health care measures into three major domains: structure, process, and outcome. Furthermore, in his article on quality he described the seven pillars of health care quality: efficacy, effectiveness, efficiency, optimality, acceptability, legitimacy, and equity.[13,14]

The work and findings of these regulatory and research agencies have led to numerous initiatives and changes that target the improvement of clinical and laboratory services in health care organizations.

Patient Safety Initiatives

Given the thousands of near misses every day and the many adverse events leading to injury, disability, and death, various initiatives have been implemented by many health care agencies, including the AHRQ and the National Patient Safety Foundation. Proposed initiatives to improve the culture of safety must take into account the following:
- Health care is a high-risk endeavor.
- Estimates on patient harm may be incorrect or underrepresented because of the methodologies used to collect the data.
- Patient health information is incomplete with the slow phase-in of electronic medical records because some hospitals only have inpatient admissions in their electronic medical record, while others only have outpatient admissions.
- Detection and analyses of adverse events and near misses should be an organizational commitment.
- A nonpunitive reporting environment that balances event reporting with disciplinary actions is ideal.[7,8,12]

Past initiatives include the National Patient Safety Goals by The Joint Commission, the Patient Safety Improvement Corp by AHRQ and Veterans Affairs, and Never Events by National Quality Forum (NQF). These initiatives vary in focus. Some focus on the reduction of events that lead to medical errors, others on the creation of assessment tools to reduce errors, and others on the establishment of standards for the provision of safe and high-quality health care. For example, in 2003, the NQF suggested 30 safe practices that would reduce error if implemented in clinical care settings. In 2006, for each safe practice, the NQF provided implementation approaches and measures for assessing the practice.

A shortcoming of many of these initiatives is the focus on clinical practice improvement and not on the improvement of laboratory services within the context of clinical medicine. In addition, in managed health care settings, laboratory medicine is often an afterthought because it contributes far less than 5% of total health care costs.[10] However, a change of focus must occur because laboratory medicine is deeply intertwined with clinical practice in the provision of quality health care. Even in managed health care settings, laboratory medicine plays a crucial role in ensuring that the appropriate care is provided at the appropriate time and setting. Furthermore, high-quality health care requires that the services rendered are cost effective and that effective management controls are in place. The Centers for Disease Control and Prevention (CDC) conceptualized and promulgated the "total testing process," a cyclical process for assessing the quality of laboratory services.[6] Among issues identified is the lack of standardization within laboratories in their request for patient-specific information. Inadequate collection of historical clinical information can lead to inappropriate interpretation of laboratory findings. In addition, preanalytic variables and postanalytic variables can significantly impact the overall quality of laboratory services, leading to erroneous laboratory results or inappropriate interpretation of reported results. Medicine is not practiced in a vacuum, and given the complexity of health care, it is important to note that all phases along the laboratory testing continuum provide opportunities for improvement, similar to other clinical services.[15] Examples by organizations that include laboratory services in their guidelines include the AHRQ's *20 Tips to Help Prevent Medical Errors,* in which patients are asked to become partners in their own health care safety by asking for their test results.[16] Another initiative that focused on

Introduction

patient safety put forth by the The Joint Commission is the National Patient Safety Goals. These include using at least two patient identifiers and emphasize timely delivery of critical test results to the appropriate clinical personnel.[17]

Although often taken for granted by many organizations, laboratory services have played a long-standing role in the provision of quality patient care. Since the 1940s, laboratories across the United States have examined their work processes and have reduced errors through appropriate training of qualified personnel, instituting quality control procedures for analytic testing and encouraging voluntary proficiency testing programs. Assessments of laboratory quality show that patient safety enhancements occur with the following system changes:

- Evaluation of individual errors as system failures
- Creation of a just culture and not a punitive one
- Increase in transparency for errors and operations
- Patient-centered and not provider-centered care
- Teamwork focus
- Increased accountability by all health care team members[3,18]

The provision of high-quality health care also includes garnering support from all levels of the organization and active involvement on the part of these individuals. Patient safety needs to be a priority from the top down. The executive team must provide training and support for those who interact with patients. In order for the multidisciplinary care teams to be effective in reducing risk, they need to have the knowledge and tools to implement strategies that will work.[19] The safety culture improvement employs the "just culture" contextual model, which requires individuals to be held accountable for mistakes but are not blamed for them.[19] By facilitating better communication and teamwork among health care providers, this model helps to improve patient safety.

References

1. Sunderman FW Sr. The history of proficiency testing/quality control. *Clin Chem.* 1992;38:1205-1209; discussion, 1218-1225.
2. Rodriquez F, Ball J. The American Society for Clinical Pathology: the pathology society of "firsts." *Lab Med.* 2007;38:596-601.
3. Leape LL. Errors in medicine. *Clin Chim Acta.* 2009;404:2-5.
4. Abdollahi A, Saffar H, Saffar H. Types and frequency of errors during different phases of testing at a clinical medical laboratory of a teaching hospital in Tehran, Iran. *N Am J Med Sci.* 2014;6:224-228.
5. Leape LL, Brennan TA, Laird N, et al. The nature of adverse events in hospitalized patients: results of the Harvard Medical Practice Study II. *N Engl J Med.* 1991;324:377-384.
6. Silverstein MD. An approach to medical errors and patient safety in laboratory services: a white paper. ResearchGate. https://www.researchgate.net/publication/237739475_An_Approach_to_Medical_Errors_and_Patient_Safety_in_Laboratory_Services_A_White_Paper_Prepared_for_the_Quality_Institute_Meeting_Making_the_Laboratory_a_Partner_in_Patient_Safety_Atlanta_April_2003_Division_of_Laboratory_Systems_Centers_for_Disease_Control_and_Prevention. Published April 2003. Accessed November 22, 2016.
7. Balogh EP, Miller BT, Ball JR, eds; Committee on Diagnostic Error in Health Care; Board on Health Care Services; Institute of Medicine; The National Academies of Sciences, Engineering, and Medicine. *Improving Diagnosis in Health Care.* Washington, DC: The National Academies Press; 2015.
8. Kohn LT, Corrigan JM, Donaldson MS, eds; Committee on Quality of Health Care in America; Institute of Medicine. *To Err is Human: Building a Safer Health System.* Washington, DC: National Academy Press; 2000.
9. Plebani M. Exploring the iceberg of errors in laboratory medicine. *Clin Chim Acta.* 2009;404:16-23.
10. Forsman RW. Why is the laboratory an afterthought for managed care organizations? *Clin Chem.* 1996;42:813-816.
11. Brennan TA, Leape LL, Laird NM, et al. Incidence of adverse events and negligence in hospitalized patients: results of the Harvard Medical Practice Study I. *N Engl J Med.* 1991;324:370-376.
12. Richardson WC, Berwick DM, Bisgard JC, eds; Committee on Quality of Health Care in America; Institute of Medicine. *Crossing the Quality Chasm: A New Health System for the 21st Century.* Washington, DC: National Academy Press; 2001.
13. Nicolay CR, Purkayastha S, Greenhalgh A, et al. Systematic review of the application of quality improvement methodologies from the manufacturing industry to surgical healthcare. *Br J Surg.* 2012;99:324-335.
14. Donabedian A. The seven pillars of quality. *Arch Pathol Lab Med.* 1990;114:1115-1118.
15. Hilborne LH, Lubin IM, Scheuner MT. The beginning of the second decade of the era of patient safety: implications and roles for the clinical laboratory and laboratory professionals. *Clin Chim Acta.* 2009;404:24-27.
16. Agency for Healthcare Research and Quality. *20 Tips to Help Prevent Medical Errors.* Rockville, MD: Agency for Healthcare Research and Quality, US Department of Health and Human Services; 2011. AHRQ publication 11-0089.
17. *2016 National Patient Safety Goals.* Oakbrook Terrace, IL: The Joint Commission; 2016.
18. Plebani M. Errors in clinical laboratories or errors in laboratory medicine? *Clin Chem Lab Med.* 2006;44:750-759.
19. Frush KS. Fundamentals of a patient safety program. *Pediatr Radiol.* 2008;38(Suppl 4):S685-S689.

2

The Culture of Patient Safety in the Laboratory

Frederick L. Kiechle, MD, PhD

Introduction

The World Health Organization defines patient safety as "the prevention of errors and adverse effects to patients that are associated with health care."[1] The safety culture and climate must be strong and supported by hospital administration to successfully achieve its patient safety goals.[1-8] The safety culture of a hospital is "the product of individual and group beliefs, values, attitudes, perceptions, competencies, and patterns of behavior that determine the organization's commitment to quality and patient safety."[1] The climate of patient safety is a window through which an organization's culture can be analyzed.[3] Climate reflects employees' perceptions of procedures, practices, and behaviors that are supported in relationship to patient safety.[3] Tests have been developed and administered worldwide to evaluate the culture of patient safety in various sections or clinical units within hospitals.[2-4,7,8] Various work areas within hospitals have been found to have quite different scores related to their perceptions of the culture of patient safety in their specific domains.[2-4,7] Over the period of 2005 to 2011, adverse event rates decreased from 5.0% to 3.7% for patients with acute myocardial infarction and from 3.7% to 2.7% for patients with congestive heart failure, while those hospitalized for pneumonia or conditions requiring surgery had no significant decline in adverse event rates.[7] Therefore, medical errors associated with some diagnostic groups have improved with time while others have not changed. Two major obstacles slowing progress in this field are availability of appropriate data and variability or different styles in the clinical practice of medicine.[2,9,10] Only 3% of data collected by more than 150 government-funded registries monitoring patient outcomes is available to the public.[10] A study from 2013 reported there were about 210,000 unintentional deaths related to medical errors in the US that year that are not reported by the Centers for Disease Control and Prevention.[10] That would place unintentional deaths related to medical errors as the third leading cause of death, just below heart disease and cancer at approximately 600,000 each in 2013.[10] The issue of prevention is as complex as the risk factors associated with medical, medication, and laboratory errors in eight countries, which include patient's age, level of education, chronic conditions, prescription drug use, the number of physicians seen, provider communication, care coordination, and emergency room visits.[11] The patient may contribute to errors in the preconsultation, consultation, or post-consultation phase of care.[12] These patient errors, like refusal to get laboratory tests drawn and performed, can lead to patient harm and medical errors.

One of the indisputable solutions to reducing hospital infection rate is the successful implementation of appropriate handwashing policies.[13] In the management of many medical errors, sunlight may be the best disinfectant.[2] In New York state, Dr Mark Chassin started reporting coronary artery bypass graft outcomes in 2009, which resulted in statewide improvement.[2] This practice instilled a sense of accountability for these data from hospital to hospital by shining a light on specific patient outcomes that reflect on the quality and safety practices of that hospital. "I've never seen hospital administrators move as fast as they do when their public image needs repair."[2]

Every section of a hospital has differences in patient volume throughout the day. Hospital leaders may react to these flow fluctuations in three ways: (1) have adequate staff at all times to accommodate the peaks, (2) intentionally staff for below-peak patient volumes and just tolerate periods of inadequate care, or (3) establish dynamic pools of staff to fill in during the peaks.[14] In the clinical or anatomic pathology laboratory, these volume fluctuations occur every day, usually with some predictability. Each of these three management choices generates a different climate among employees. The selection of one of the three choices begins with knowing if hospital administration views the clinical and anatomic pathology laboratories as cost centers or profit centers. The inadequate staffing model (the second choice) would be selected by administrators who see the laboratory as a cost center, a necessary division that drains funds from the operating budget. Usually, inadequate staffing is associated with inadequate space and equipment. Requests for laboratory tests requiring new, disruptive innovation[15]—such as matrix-assisted laser desorption ionization time-of-flight mass spectrometry (MALDI-TOF) for the identification of bacteria,[16] next-generation sequence technology for determining drugable mutations in various cancers,[17] or use of cell-free fetal DNA

Table 2-1. Laboratory Errors Defined by Cause

	O'Kane[30]	Carraro[31]	Plebani[32]
Preanalytic	87.6%	61.9%	68.2%
Analytic	11.1%	15.0%	13.3%
Postanalytic	1.3%	23.1%	18.5%

Table 2-2. Examples of Preanalytic Errors in Clinical Pathology

Action and Potential Associated Error	Reference
1. Computer physician order entry	33
a. Inappropriate test selection	34, 35
b. Obsolete test selection	15, 34, 35
c. Duplicate order	36
d. Test ordered in error	
2. Patient preparation	29
3. Phlebotomy	37, 40
a. Specimen unlabeled → rejected	29
b. Specimen mislabeled	29, 38, 41, 42
c. Wrist band	41, 43, 44
i. Absent	
ii. Inaccurate	
d. Specimen collection	29, 37
i. Collected from infusion site	37
ii. Inadequate specimen: anticoagulant ratio → rejected	39
iii. Hemolysis, icterus, lipemia	29, 45, 46
iv. Mismatched requisition and label	41
v. Test timing error (eg, therapeutic drug monitoring)	29
vi. Specimen clotted → rejected	39
vii. Wrong anticoagulant	29
e. Specimen transport	
i. Temperature (room temperature, on ice, frozen)	29
ii. Drones	47
iii. Pneumatic tube	48
iv. Specimen damaged	29

in maternal blood circulation for detection of trisomy 21[18]—would be sent out to a reference laboratory.[19,20] The inadequate staffing creates inefficiency and stress, which leads to laboratory errors such as failure to call critical values, delays in turnaround time for stat tests, failure to add tests to existing orders, and so forth. Incident reports are followed by root cause analysis,[21] which generates a crisis management response from administrators, who leave their offices and visit the laboratories, doing the leadership walk-arounds asking patient safety questions that may have prevented the crisis in the first place.[2,22-24] Complacency[23] and unaccountability[2,24] are much more common than we perceive because these issues can be invisible to the people involved. Short-term or long-term financial "success easily produces complacency."[23] There are some issues that require a response with a sense of urgency because the problem is of pressing importance to improve patient safety.

Returning to our three choices for solving fluctuating test volumes, the first and third choices would be preferred by hospital administrators who view the laboratory as a profit center. Often this goal is achieved by expanding the core laboratory business serving registered outpatients and inpatients to serving non-patients from physician offices, nursing homes, or other hospitals.[25] This outreach laboratory will increase the volume of current tests on the menu and increase esoteric test volumes to a point where they are profitable to bring in house from the reference laboratory. Increased test volume will reduce the unit cost per test, maximizing the laboratory component of a diagnosis-related group lump sum and capitated laboratory contracts with a price per member per month (PMPM).[25] The outreach program should be structured so that the usual number of administrators required to sign off on purchases, rental spaces, and contracts is reduced to two or three individuals only. This streamlining assures easy mobilization of a sense of urgency required to meet the competition's activity in the market place.[25] The attentiveness to client satisfaction usually creates a positive climate and culture for patient safety in this setting.

The remainder of this chapter will focus on errors that have been reported in clinical and anatomic pathology and potential strategic solutions.

Classification of Errors in Clinical Pathology

Because 80% to 90% of all diagnoses are made using laboratory test results, clearly laboratory errors will have a major impact on patient care.[6,26] From 1986 to 2002, the error rates in a variety of clinical diagnostic laboratories worldwide varied from 0.08% to 9.36%.[6] These errors have been divided into preanalytic, analytic, and postanalytic.[6,27-29] Table 2-1 demonstrates the variability in the distribution of errors in these three categories.[30-32] Generally, preanalytic and postanalytic errors are greater than analytic errors.[26]

Preanalytic Errors in Clinical Pathology

Table 2-2 lists a variety of examples of common preanalytic errors.[15,29,33-48] The majority of these errors occur outside the laboratory during the test ordering, phlebotomy, specimen collection, and specimen transportation to the laboratory (Table 2-2). Computerized order entry is more likely to be performed by a physician today. The formatting of the tests in specific order sets or in alphabetic lists may influence which test is selected.[49] The selected test may be inappropriate for the clinical question asked[34,35,50] or may be obsolete and provide little value.[15,35] Obsolete tests are not universally accepted as useless, and therefore manufacturers may continue to make the reagents and reference laboratories will continue to offer them if they are ordered by physicians.[15] This creates a "leak" in the laboratory test formulary.[51] The inability to eliminate the availability of obsolete laboratory tests increases the potential for interpretation errors of laboratory results (postanalytic errors).

Patient preparation is also important. Overnight fasting is necessary to obtain accurate fasting blood glucose for evaluation of potential diabetes mellitus. Timing of the collection of a blood specimen for a peak or trough drug level after a specific time after the last drug dose is essential. A well-trained phlebotomist will provide the best quality blood specimens. Often the staff performing this service is no longer under the jurisdiction of the laboratory leadership. Attempts to provide adequate training to nurses, nursing aides, respiratory therapists, and other nonlaboratorians can be very challenging. Bad practices can become institutionalized, resulting in blood specimens with a high degree of hemolysis that may need to be rejected by the laboratory and redrawn. The frequency of hemolysis varies with the degree of phlebotomy training and the method used to collect the blood specimen. The range of hemolyzed samples varies in the literature from 3.8% for a 21-gauge needle into a vacuum specimen collection tube to 100% when a 24-gauge intravenous catheter is used.[52] The gauge of the needle is inversely proportional to the diameter, so the higher the gauge the smaller the diameter of the needle.[53] A needle of 24-gauge or greater will cause lysis of red blood cells as they travel under extreme shear stress through the small bore of the needle. Not all laboratory tests are altered to the same degree by the presence of hemolysis.[54] The presence of 1% hemolyzed red blood cells may result in one of four categories of degree of change, depending on the analyte measured: seriously affected (>100%; aspartate aminotransferase [AST], lactate dehydrogenase [LD], potassium [K]); noticeably affected (20%-99%, alanine aminotransferase [ALT], iron, thyroxine [T4]); slightly affected (1%-19%); or not affected.[54] In a review of 772 laboratories, the hemolysis rate varied from less than 1% to greater than 15%.[55] Visual inspection is an unreliable method to assess hemolysis, but it is used by 48% of the laboratories.[55] Instrument-calculated hemolytic index scales are less subjective and provide reproducible values from 1 to 8, from which appropriate hemolysis-effect computer comments can be generated.[46,56] In whole blood specimens, hemolysis can only be detected after centrifugation of the specimen and visualization of the plasma.[55] Hemolysis is usually caused by poor phlebotomy practices, a preanalytic error that may create potential analytic errors in the measurement of specific analytes, which may lead to diagnostic clinical errors such as false increases or decreases.[54,55]

A misidentified specimen may lead to the release of results to the wrong patient. In a review of 120 laboratories, 85.5% of identification errors were detected before verification of the results, while the remaining 14.5% were detected after the results were released.[41] Mislabeling errors may be identified before verification by blood type mismatch with historical patient blood type, delta checks using mean red blood cell volume (MCV)[57] or logical complete blood count delta check,[58] or using optical character recognition to compare the patient's name in the laboratory information system (LIS) with the patient's name printed on the customer's label.[42] The latter system failed to identify 25% of mislabeled specimens because of nonstandard fonts, misaligned labels, or truncated names.[42] These aberrations were handled manually and need to be programmed into the system for rapid identification.

Pneumatic tube systems are used to deliver specimens to the clinical laboratories to reduce turnaround time. Because it takes up to an hour for most whole blood specimens to clot in nonanticoagulated collection tubes, the majority of specimens sent through a pneumatic tube system will be unclotted when they arrive at the laboratory. To reduce the chance of damaging the cellular components in whole blood, a soft-land cushion decelerates the pneumatic carriers as they approach the laboratory and gently drops them into the receiving area[48]; however, the mechanical disruption can cause hemolysis,[59] and the disruption of white cells from patients with leukemia may result in pseudohyperkalemia.[60] Phlebotomists can prevent air bubbles from developing in heparinized whole blood, which create perturbations in PO_2 values, by placing the specimen in a pressure-sealed container before sending it through the pneumatic tube.[61] An alternative transport device may be an unmanned aerial system or drone,[47] which has the advantage of avoiding traffic delays and covering long distances. Blood specimens for chemistry, hematology, and coagulation were flown from 6 to 38 minutes in a drone at 76°F or 79°F and were tested with duplicate tubes not flown in a drone. Only bicarbonate failed to meet the allowable limits criteria.[47]

After the specimen arrives safely at the laboratory, there are still a few preanalytic processes to complete: (1) accessioning the specimen using the LIS, (2) sorting the tubes by testing location, (3) aliquotting volumes from a parent tube to a daughter tube for a second testing location, and (4) decapping the tube if cork-piercing technology is not available. These processes may be done manually or using automated preanalytic components.[6,62,63] The first component is a batch input module that accepts capped tubes, reads their barcode labels, and accessions them into the LIS.[62,63] Next, the tubes can be sorted or sent directly to an automatic balancing centrifuge. After centrifugation, the tubes may be decapped, if required, and sent down a track to the analyzer located adjacent to this track.[62,63] This automation eliminates numerous manual steps that are a common source of laboratory errors.[6,62]

The majority of laboratory errors occur in the preanalytic phase, and care must be taken to evaluate and minimize the frequency of these occurrences to avoid downstream diagnostic errors.[64,65]

Analytic Errors in Clinical Pathology

Analytic errors should be evaluated related to the functions and features of the type of quantitative analyzers that are used in a laboratory[29,66-75] (Table 2-3). Falsely low sodium (pseudohyponatremia), pseudonormonatremia, or suppressed physiologically increased sodium can occur in serum or plasma specimens with hyperlipidemia or hyperproteinemia.[66-68] This error occurs in high-throughput analyzers that use indirect potentiometry to measure sodium. This method requires a specimen dilution step before measurement, which, in the presence of high levels of lipid or protein, will decrease the sodium measured in the water concentration.[66-68] This result places the patient at risk for inappropriate therapeutic intervention or lack of it. To substantiate the presence of this artifact, sodium measurement should be performed using direct potentiometry, which does not dilute the specimen before its measurement.[66,68]

Because many automated laboratory analyzers can be accessed remotely through a hospital's network, they are vulnerable to hackers who could change reference ranges or other parameters and create artificial medical emergencies or therapeutic misadventures. In a related issue, the Food and Drug Administration (FDA), the US Department of Homeland Security Industrial Control Systems Cyber Emergency Response Team, and Hospira have reported the cybersecurity vulnerabilities associated with the Symbiq Infusion System (Hospira; Lake Forest, IL).[69] Low-skilled hackers could control the device and alter the drug dosage infused into the patient.[69] Theoretically, this event could occur with laboratory analyzers linked to vendors through networks.

Reagent carryover may occur in automated analyzers when reagent clings to a pipette tip that moves from one specimen assay setup to the next or when unclean, reusable cuvettes with reagent residue left behind are used.[70] These issues may result in reports that are falsely low or falsely high.[70] Specimen carryover may be an issue as well, where a high quantitative result, such as for human chorionic gonadotropin, is carried over to a very low-value specimen.[76] Protocols need to be developed for the detection of reagent or specimen carryover.[70,76]

When new quantitative analyzers are introduced—and periodically thereafter—calibration, calibration verification, linearity, and verification of the analytic measurements range is required.[71] The analytic measurement range is usually greater than the reference range for an analyte.[77] Quality control is performed based on Westgard rules.[72] The analyzer's software (middleware or LIS) should have rules that alert the analyzer operator of an out-of-range error.[72] This issue needs immediate attention before further specimens are analyzed. Repeating the quality control run or performing analyzer maintenance may be required to remedy the problem. If the run of specimens is permitted to continue after a quality control failure, all of the subsequent results need to be reviewed for accuracy and usually will need to be repeated. Analyzers may cause random errors[29]; these errors may be detected as critical values or during delta check reviews.[58]

Frozen specimens must be thawed before they can be analyzed. Frozen specimens may be subject to freeze-thaw cycles when stored at -20°C in frost-free freezers.[73] Using insulated containers may help prevent thawing during these cycles. In general, frozen

Table 2-3. Examples of Analytic Errors in Clinical Pathology	
Action and Potential Associated Error	**Reference**
1. Equipment malfunction	29
a. Hypernatremia/pseudonormonatremia	66-68
b. Hacking	69
c. Reagent carryover	70
2. Error in verifying performance of quantitative analytic systems	71
3. Undetected failure in quality control	29, 72
4. Instrument-caused random error	29
5. Frozen specimen thawing	73, 74
6. Centrifuge brake and coagulation results	75

serum or plasma specimens should be thawed at room temperature; rapid thawing using heat may result in decomposition of components. To disrupt concentration gradients during thawing, the sample should be inverted 10 to 20 times.[74] If undissolved material is present, controlled warming may bring the particles into solution. An automated workcell for thawing 760 specimens has been reported.[74] Frozen specimens are placed in racks with an opening at the bottom that allows room temperature air to circulate, thawing specimens in 22 to 23 minutes. Specimens are inverted 8 times with an automated arm.[74]

Centrifuges, either stand alone or incorporated into an automated preanalytic module,[62,63,78] usually have an option for braking at the end or not.[75] Centrifuge braking reduces the total time for the centrifugation process. Centrifugation of whole, anticoagulated blood samples is necessary to generate platelet-poor plasma with a residual platelet count of less than 10×10^9/L.[75] Daves et al[75] have demonstrated that the platelet count in platelet-poor plasma is higher, prothrombin time is prolonged, and fibrinogen is significantly higher with the brake on compared with the brake off during centrifugation of coagulation test specimens. The quality of platelet-poor plasma generated after centrifugation should always be checked on a routine basis to assure adequate quality for routine coagulation test performance.

There are numerous processes involved in the analytic phase of laboratory testing. Each process is a potential source of error and should be assessed according to the functions and features of the analytic system in use.

Postanalytic Errors in Clinical Pathology

This phase is dependent on communication between laboratory staff and clinicians.[27] Table 2-4 provides a list of potential postanalytic errors in the clinical laboratory.[26-29,79-84] Critical values or "panic values" are established to identify laboratory test results that require immediate notification of the health care team caring for a patient whose laboratory results suggest that a rapid therapeutic intervention is required for the patient to survive.[26] These values need to be called to the appropriate individual on the nursing unit were the patient is located. If no one is available to take the call, repeated calling is required until someone is reached. If no one responds after a specific time interval, there should be a policy for who should be called in nursing or physician administration to relay the information.

Errors in manual data entry of laboratory results or other computer-related errors may lead to issuing an incorrect laboratory result to a patient.[29] These errors may be identified within the laboratory using delta checks[57,58] or other methods, or by the physician or

Table 2-4. Examples of Postanalytic Errors in Clinical Pathology

Action and Potential Associated Error	Reference
1. Results reporting	29
a. Critical value reporting	26-28
b. Improper data entry; results reported incorrectly	29
c. Reported to wrong provider	29
d. Delay in reporting results	27-29, 79
2. Results misinterpreted	27, 28
a. Reference range variability (age, sex, transgender)	80-83
b. Data integrity failures in electronic health records	84
c. Neglecting change management for networked device or systems	84
3. Failure to act on results	29

nurse who questions the accuracy of the result. A protocol should be available for how to evaluate these issues in a systematic manner. Usually a quality systems team member would be called in to assist.

Some delays in reporting results[27-29,79] are unavoidable, such as LIS failures, analyzer maintenance, specimen transport failures, staffing shortages, and others. If these events are planned or unplanned and will be of long duration (more than 1 hour), the situation needs to be communicated throughout the hospital. If the LIS will be down for more than 1 hour, a protocol-defined paper requisition backup plan needs to be activated. Delays in receipt of reference laboratory results may be related to weather or to failure of internal processes. In either case, the reference laboratory must communicate these issues to its clients in real time.

The misinterpretation of laboratory results by the ordering physician is always a possible source of postanalytic error.[27,28] Interpretation comments attached to specific test results may be useful and should be used often. For example, urine screens by immunoassay for drugs of abuse need comments for each drug family that define the positive cutoff value, which drugs in the family will be positive or negative, or drugs that may result in a false-positive reaction.[85] Molecular assays for viral load (eg, human immunodeficiency virus [HIV], hepatitis C virus [HCV]) need to have the lower limit of detection defined in the comment. These comments, to remain useful, need to be reviewed whenever a new method is introduced, or at least annually, for accuracy.

Interpretation of laboratory results and subsequent decision making are based on reference intervals.

Procedures for transfer and validation of reference intervals should be established in every clinical laboratory.[77] There are many analytes that require age-specific reference ranges.[80-81] These ranges need to be evaluated at the time of new test introduction and periodically thereafter.

The greatest barrier to transgender medical care is the lack of knowledgeable providers.[82,86] Transgender men (female to male) are treated with testosterone to achieve a normal male physiologic range (30-1000 ng/dL or 1.04-34.7 nmol/L). Transgender women (male to female) are treated with antiandrogen and estrogen to decrease testosterone levels to normal female physiologic range (30-100 ng/dL or 1.04-3.47 nmol/L) without excessive estradiol levels (<200 pg/mL or <734.2 pmol/L).[82] Transgender women's laboratory values were compared with those of 20 male and 20 female nontransgender individuals.[83] Hemoglobin, hematocrit, and low-density lipoprotein resembled female values, while alkaline phosphatase, potassium, and creatinine resembled male values.[83] These results suggest that new reference intervals are required during the transgender transition process and at the final outcome.

The ECRI Institute has published a "top 10 list" of technology safety hazards along with risk mitigation strategies.[84] Two of the safety hazards are applicable to clinical pathology. The first safety hazard is data integrity failures in electronic health records and other health information technology systems.[84] The integrity of data within a system and shared with other systems must be ensured in order to avoid inappropriate treatment. Examples cited include "patient data from a medical device or system mistakenly being associated with another patient's record, clock synchronization errors, or inappropriate use of default values."[84] The second safety hazard is neglecting change management for networked devices and systems. Any change in software or wireless networks may lead to unanticipated loss or defects in downstream processes.[84]

Finally, the failure to act on abnormal laboratory results is a very common and unfortunate source of postanalytic error.[29] If the abnormal laboratory value reaches a panic/critical value, it will be called within 5 minutes or less to the appropriate health care team member taking care of the patient. However, if a laboratory test is ordered by a physician, it is assumed that it will be reviewed by that individual within a reasonable time after the result is available. For example, a patient with chest pain and a normal troponin I may be having a myocardial infarction, reflected by an increased troponin I after the next specimen is drawn after 3 hours. If this value is not noted by anyone on the floor, the outcome may be fatal hours later. The laboratory has limited staff and cannot be asked to call about every potentially high-risk laboratory result. The system requires accountability at both ends—the laboratory and the ordering physician—to avoid unnecessary, missed, clinically significant laboratory results, such as slowly increasing white blood count during developing sepsis.

Point-of-Care Testing

Point-of-care testing (POCT) is laboratory testing performed at or near the patient's bedside, and the results are used for diagnostic or therapeutic decisions.[87] The Clinical Laboratory Improvement Amendments of 1988 (CLIA '88) tests may be waived, provider-performed microscopy, or moderately complex.[87-95] There are a large variety of CLIA tests that have been classified as waived by the FDA, and a list of them from 2000 to the present can be found at www.accessdata.fda.gov/scripts/cdrh/cfdocs/cfclia/testswaived.cfm (accessed Nov 2016). Just like highly complex laboratory tests previously discussed, POCT must be evaluated and improved after reviewing the total testing process—preanalytic, analytic, and postanalytic phases.[87,96-99] Error rates in these three phases are rarely reported. O'Kane et al[99] reported more analytic errors than preanalytic errors when POCT was compared with testing performed in the central laboratory; however, preanalytic errors outnumbered analytic errors in a similar study done in a neonatal intensive care unit.[97] In a survey of 111 general practices in the Netherlands using POCT, preanalytic and analytic errors occurred at about the same frequency.[96]

There are at least 14 different sources of body fluids in a human.[92] Point-of-care analysis has been limited to urinalysis by dipstick[92] and a variety of labile specimens examined under a bright field or a phase contrast microscope, which are classified as provider-performed microscopy by CLIA '88.[94,95] These assays may be performed after obtaining a separate license from Centers for Medicare and Medicaid Services (CMS). These assays include KOH preparation, pinworm detection, fern test, microscopic urinalysis, semen analysis for presence of sperm and motility, and detection of eosinophils in nasal smears.[94,95] The potential for errors exists when off-label use of blood tests—for example, a glucose oxidase strip for detection of cerebrospinal fluid (CSF) versus nasal discharge[100] or a reagent urine dipstick for detection of bacterial contamination of platelet concentrate[101,102]—occurs with a body fluid in the absence of a commercially available product designed for the specific clinical situation. The use of glucose oxidase reagent blood strips is an unreliable method for detecting CSF rhinorrhea or drainage from the ear. The CSF leakage may be secondary to a congenital defect or head trauma. Every laboratory supporting a level 1 trauma center should have a method validated to distinguish CSF from nasal secretions and/or blood: detection of β2-transferrin or beta-trace protein.[92,103] Bacterial contamination of platelet concentrates occurs in 1/1000 to 1/3000 units transfused.[102] The most successful method would have a high sensitivity and specificity, and be reliable, inexpensive, and fast. Currently, there is no method available that fits all of those criteria. However, methods that are performed at the point-of-issue seem the most likely to be successful. An early method measured glucose and pH using a urine dipstick and has been abandoned secondary to a high false-positive rate.[101,102] Other methods are under development.[102]

As a paradigm to waived POCT in a hospital and issues related to patient safety, let's look at glucose, the most common hospital-based POCT test. Table 2-5 lists examples of errors that may occur in glucose POCT.[37,91,104-113] Glucose POCT devices may use capillary, venous, or arterial blood. Three detection methods are common: glucose oxidase, glucose dehydrogenase, or hexokinase.[113] Roche (Indianapolis, IN) uses a mutant variant of the quinoprotein glucose dehydrogenase enzyme to improve D-glucose sensitivity; minimize inference from maltose galactose, triglycerides, ascorbic acid, and acetaminophen[106,111]; and eliminate errors caused by high and low oxygen concentrations.[106] Hypotension, defined as systolic blood pressure less than 80 mm Hg, will cause falsely decreased capillary glucose measurements because the specimen is primarily interstitial fluid, secondary to the blood retreating to the central organs to keep them functioning.[105,106,113]

There is an ongoing debate related to the safety of using waived glucose meters to measure glucose in critically ill patients.[107,112] At a public meeting held by the FDA, entitled Clinical Accuracy Requirements for Point-of-Care Blood Glucose Meters, on March 16-17, 2010, it was implied that there may be a need for two types of glucose meters: one for home use and another with greater precision for hospital use. This desire was reflected in FDA-required language in glucose strip packaging literature stating that these strips and glucose meters should not be used in critically ill patients[114]; however, neither CMS nor the FDA has defined a critically ill patient.[114] Using the glucose meter and glucose strips in critically ill patients represents an off-label use that converts the waived test to highly complex test and decertifies most of the waived testers. Efforts have been made to validate specific glucose meters for use in critically ill patients.[107] This patient population is more likely to have fluctuations in blood pressure[105,106,113] and PO_2[106]; to have edema[109] or dehydration; and to be taking medications such as dopamine, which interferes with glucose dehydrogenase

Table 2-5. Examples of Errors in Glucose Point-of-Care Testing

Action and Potential Associated Error	Reference
Preanalytic	
1. Specimen collection	
a. Bad fingerstick technique	37, 104, 107
b. Hypotension or shock	105, 106, 113
c. Dehydration	
d. Edema	107, 109
e. Failure to let alcohol dry	37
f. Improper dosing of test strip	106
g. Temperature extremes	91, 106
h. Improper specimen type (capillary vs venous vs arterial)	109, 112, 113
2. Patient identification	108
Analytic	
1. Hematocrit effect	110, 111, 113
2. Medication interference	106, 107, 111, 113
3. pH, O_2 or CO_2 tension	106
4. Incorrect calibration	113
5. Operator error	106, 113
Postanalytic	
1. Interface transmission of results error	113

results, or ascorbic acid and acetaminophen, which interfere with glucose oxidase results.[106,113] Critically ill children have a U-shaped relationship between early blood glucose concentration (<65 mg/dL [3.6 mmol/L] and >200 mg/dL [11.1 mmol/L]) and mortality.[115] A group of critical care medicine physicians published consensus recommendations for critically ill patients.[112] If the patient requires invasive vascular monitoring with an arterial line or, second best, a venous line for glucose blood specimens, capillary specimens are inaccurate and should not be used.[112] If invasive vascular monitoring is not required, then capillary specimens may be used. The type of blood specimen should be recorded for each blood glucose measured. This dialogue continues, while hospital laboratories struggle with their definition—and then validation—of their old, waived glucose meters to use in critically ill patients. Meanwhile, exclusion of these patients from waived point-of-care glucose testing will lead to patient safety concerns, including increased glucose turnaround time, delayed therapeutic decision on insulin dose regulation, and others.

Classification of Errors in Anatomic Pathology

Anatomic pathology in a hospital is subdivided into surgical pathology, cytology, and the autopsy service. The activities in these three subdivisions are similar and can be divided into the usual workflow of three basic phases: preanalytic, analytic, and postanalytic[115-131] (Table 2-6). In a review of medical malpractice lawsuits related to pathology, the most common issue was the alleged missed diagnosis of melanoma, followed by breast biopsies, gynecologic specimens, and preanalytic errors.[124] False-negative Papanicolaou smears (37/48 cases) were the most common cytology issues. Transfusion-acquired HIV infection was the most common clinical pathology issue (32/36 cases).[124] Preanalytic surgical specimen identification errors are a source of potential patient safety problems related to the wrong patient receiving another patient's diagnosis.[116] A 3-month study of these errors in 69 hospitals revealed 2.9% identification defects, 1.2% container defects, and 2.3% requisition defects.[125] Another study reviewed mislabeled specimens in anatomic pathology over an 18-month period.[122] They identified 75 errors (0.25% of cases), with 73% involving patient name and 24% involving site.[122] The gross room was the source of 69% of these two errors, and 73% of these errors resulted in slides assigned to an incorrect patient.[122] These errors combined with misinterpretations and pathology report defects resulted in 4.8/1000 to 10/1000 amended surgical pathology reports.[131] Report defects may be related to workload.[121] The relationship between workload and diagnostic error rates may be bimodal, in that higher error rates occur with low workload due to inexperience and with high workload due to lack of time for thorough evaluation.[121]

A request for a second-opinion review of a difficult surgical pathology case will reduce errors.[117,119,123,127,130] Subspecialty pathologic review of the original slides in cancer cases before initiation of treatment revealed agreement in 75% of 2718 cases, minor discrepancies in 18.7%, and change in diagnosis in 6.2% of cases.[123] Breast pathology, for example, generates frequent second-opinion requests based on laboratory policies focused on diagnosis[127]: invasive cancer, 65%; ductal carcinoma in situ, 56%; and atypical ductal hyperplasia, 36%. Agreement between the original report and the second opinion is dependent on the diagnosis.[130] The worst agreement occurs with columnar cell lesions without atypia and pleomorphic lobular carcinoma in situ.[131] Tissues or cells may contaminate surgical or cytology specimens secondary to floaters from another case in the histologist's water bath.[129] Tissue from males versus females may be determined using molecular techniques to identify two X chromosomes versus an X and a Y chromosome in the adjacent tissues or cells.[129] DNA polymorphisms comparing allelic patterns may be used to distinguish two female or two male tissue samples or cells from each other.[129] Surgical pathology defect rates have been evaluated by the College of American Pathologists (CAP) Q-Probes program.[132] It was found that misinterpretations and specimen defects were most often detected by pathologists, whereas misidentifications were most often detected by clinicians.[132]

Monitoring Errors in Clinical and Anatomic Pathology

The total testing process in both clinical and anatomic pathology involves the same three phases: preanalytic, analytic, and postanalytic. Errors can occur at any point in this total testing process. A pathology quality improvement program usually consists of a variety of quality indicators or metrics that are used to monitor and improve the quality of service.[28,133,134] The assumption is that "quality cannot be improved without

Table 2-6. Examples of Errors in Anatomic Pathology	
Action and Potential Associated Errors	**Reference**
Preanalytic	
1. Specimen identification errors	
a. Tracking with barcodes	120, 126
b. Patient identification	122, 125, 128
c. Specimen source	122, 125, 128
2. Reliable clinical information	
a. Delay in diagnosis	116
b. Amended report	116, 118, 128, 131
Analytic	
1. Gross and specimen examination	116
2. Dissection and sectioning	116
3. Histologic processing and staining	116
4. Microscopic evaluation errors	116, 124
a. Peer review	116
b. Expert's second opinion	117, 119, 123, 127, 130
c. Correlation studies	118
d. Workload	121
e. Tissue contamination	129
Postanalytic	
1. Complete reports	116
2. Critical values	116, 117

being measured."[28] It has been said that a laboratory measures what it values and values what it measures. A good quality indicator should be pertinent, reliable, practical, measurable, accurate, understandable, and effective.[28] A quality indicator should monitor the frequency of recurring errors within the laboratory and/or their effect outside the laboratory (patient outcome). They should be quantified: number of hemolyzed samples/total number of samples, expressed as a percentage.[28,133] There should be a link to potential resolutions of the problem and a benchmark frequency of the problem from the literature. If the frequency of a problem remains at the benchmark frequency or below, the quality indicators should be considered for temporary or permanent retirement. This review process keeps the quality indicators relevant to the real-time issues facing the laboratory.

The CAP has offered a comprehensive portfolio of quality indicators in clinical and anatomic pathology called the Q-Probes program.[38,41,132,135-139] Their Q-Tracks program has offered longitudinal performance monitoring of 19 quality indicators for a duration of 5 to 10 years.[26,43,135-137] These benchmarking exercises provide a source for a laboratory's quality indicator benchmark. Both Q-Probes and Q-Tracks programs have demonstrated improvement in laboratory performance over time.[26,38,41,43,132,135-139]

These programs tend to focus on laboratory efficiency and internal quality rather than on patient outcomes.[140] When establishing quality indicators, their potential consequence on patient outcome and the feasibility of measuring this effect should be evaluated. For example, if an inappropriate test is ordered, what effect would a false-positive result have on diagnostic error? It could lead to unnecessary additional workup of a nonexistent disease.

Risk management techniques and standards have found their way into the clinical laboratory via Clinical and Laboratory Standards Institute (CLSI) document EP23-A.[141] This document explains how to develop and maintain a quality control plan through identification of weaknesses (risks) in the preanalytic, analytic, and postanalytic phases of testing. From this analysis, specific actions are derived to detect, prevent, and control errors that can result in harm to the patient.[142] These tools may be useful in evaluating the risks related to potential errors in all three phases of clinical and anatomic pathology testing.

Error Reporting and Follow-Up

When departments of anatomic pathology (AP) and academic clinical pathology (CP) were asked to whom they reported medical errors, three hospital programs were revealed: incident reporting, 54.0% AP, 86% CP; risk management, 59.3% AP, 43% CP; and patient safety program, 20.7% AP.[143] The incident reporting system identifies risks so that organizations can implement interventions to reduce these risks[143-146]; the Institute of Medicine recommends its use[147] and The Joint Commission requires that all hospitals have and use it, as well as report medical errors directly to patients.[144,145] The incident reporting system cannot be used to measure error rates, to compare organizations, or to measure changes over time.[145] The primary reason is that incident reports focus on one event and under-report the actual number of similar events that occur.[145,146] To obtain a more comprehensive overview of medical errors in hospitals, investigations should combine information from multiple sources, such as incident reports, patient complaints, and retrospective chart review of deceased patients.[146] The investigation of an incident report may use root cause analysis[21] to define the risks and refine a plan to avoid a recurrence of this specific incident.

The characteristics of a good medical error reporting system include nonpunitive reporting, confidential handling of information, independence with no relationship to regulatory issues such as licensing, and a primary focus of collecting information to permit the design of more effective strategies to minimize the systems contributions to such incidents.[6] Incident reporting systems strive to incorporate these elements. This system provides some unique value when used correctly.[145] It can be used to identify local system hazards, to aggregate experience for uncommon conditions, to share lessons within and across organizations, and to increase patient safety culture.[145]

Patient safety culture encourages transparency, including disclosure of medical errors to patients.[143,144,148-151] The Joint Commission introduced a nationwide disclosure standard in 2001 that includes all outcomes of care—those anticipated and unanticipated.[152] A survey of risk managers in 2002 reported 36% of institutions had disclosure policies, which increased to 69% by 2005.[144] States have enacted disclosure-related legislation—beginning with Pennsylvania in 2002, which requires patient notification within 7 days of a serious event.[144] The University of Michigan Health System demonstrated that the introduction of a disclosure-with-offer program decreased the monthly rate of new claims and lawsuits.[153,154] Physicians do not feel comfortable with the process of admitting medical errors to a patient and/or their family.[143,144,150,151] A team approach is recommended, with the attending physician leading the conversation.[151] Premeeting preparation is important to review the details of the case. If there is any indication that surgical or cytology specimens or clinical laboratory results may have some relationship to the medical error incident, then the appropriate pathologist(s) should be included in the team.[151] Physician engagement in all aspects of the patient safety culture strengthens the success of the assimilation process.[155] "I know there's a proverb that says 'To err is human!' But a human error is nothing to what a computer can do if it tries."[156]

Just Culture: Foundation for the Laboratory Culture of Patient Safety

An important element to include in a good medical error reporting system is nonpunitive reporting.[6] Patient safety requires two key elements: system reliability and human reliability. In short, an individual should not be held accountable for mistakes made in a system they have no authority to control.[157,158] *Just culture* is defined as a learning culture where errors are viewed as opportunities to improve our understanding of risk. Just culture holds all employees responsible for the quality of their choices during an unintentional error (slips or lapses)—the employee should not be held accountable but rather should be supported and involved in the root cause analysis process. However, employees exhibiting actions that are risky, reckless, or malicious, or who exhibit impaired judgment, may require coaching and/or disciplinary action.[158] Just culture emphasizes the importance of the evaluation of system design and the management of employee behavior selections to improve patient safety, and diminishes emphasis on outcomes and errors.[157,158] Every near-miss episode is an opportunity to diminish elements of system risk and behavioral risk associated with the episode to avoid its recurrence. The origin of an unsafe act may rest within the system or organization if an individual with similar skills and background would state that they would have acted in the same manner in the same situation.[157] Just culture provides the foundation for achieving a laboratory culture of patient safety.

Two other tools work synergistically with just culture. They are teamwork training and walk rounds.[22,157] All three are optimized if they are systematically and consistently implemented in an integrated fashion. However, this implementation process is not easy, and results are difficult to measure. During walk rounds, leadership and employees engage in informal conversation where findings from recent root cause analysis can be shared and discussed. Problems related to patient safety may be revealed, and it is leadership's responsibility to resolve these issues. The solutions are then brought back to be shared with the employees, closing the circle of potential errors.[22,157]

Effective teamwork and communication must be taught and practiced at levels of administration and within each department and section of a department. These skills will assist in ongoing effective collaborative work as the health care team proceeds through their workday. Various strategies for teaching these skills have been described, and there is no standard method that fits all the complexities that various health care institutions exhibit.[157]

If these three tools—just culture, teamwork training, and walk rounds—are effectively and consistently implemented in a health care institution, the culture of patient safety will flourish and prosper.

References

1. The Joint Commission. Patient safety systems. In: *2015 Comprehensive Accreditation Manual for Hospitals*. Update 2. Oak Brook, IL: Joint Commission Resources; 2016:PS1-PS54.
2. Makary M. *Unaccountable: What Hospitals Won't Tell You and How Transparency can Revolutionize Health Care.* New York, NY: Bloomsbury Press; 2012.
3. Ginsburg LR, Tregunno D, Norton PG, Mitchell JI, Howley H. "Not another safety culture survey": using the Canadian patient safety climate survey (Can-PSCS) to measure provider perceptions of PSC across health settings. *BMJ Qual Saf.* 2014;23(2):162-170.
4. Vlayen A, Schrooten W, Wami W, et al. Variability of patient safety culture in Belgian acute hospitals. *J Patient Saf.* 2015;11(2):110-121.
5. Donaldson L. The challenge of quality and patient safety. *J R Soc Med.* 2008;101(7):338-341.
6. Kalra J. *Medical Errors and Patient Safety: Strategies to Reduce and Disclose Medical Errors and Improve Patient Safety.* Berlin, Germany: Walter de Gruyter GmbH & Co; 2011.
7. Singer SJ, Gaba DM, Falwell A, Lin S, Hayes J, Baker L. Patient safety in 92 US hospitals: differences by work area and discipline. *Med Care.* 2009;47(1):23-31.
8. Wagner C, Smits M, Sorra J, Huang CC. Assessing patient safety culture in hospitals across countries. *Int J Qual Health Care.* 2013;25(3):213-221.
9. Wang Y, Eldridge N, Metersky ML, et al. National trends in patient safety for four common conditions, 2005 – 2011. *N Engl J Med.* 2014;370(4):341-351.
10. Makary MA, Daniel M. Medical error: the third leading cause of death in the US. *BMJ.* 2016;353:i2139.
11. Scobie A. Self-reported medical, medication and laboratory error in eight countries: risk factors for chronically ill adults. *Int J Qual Health Care.* 2011;22(3):182-186.
12. Buetow S, Elwyn G. Patient safety and patient error. *Lancet.* 2007;369(9556):158-161.
13. Luangasanatip N, Hongsuwan M, Limmauthurotsakul D, et al. Comparative efficiency of interventions to promote hand hygiene in hospital: systematic review and network meta-analysis. *BMJ.* 2015;351:h3728.
14. Litvak E, Fineberg HV. Smoothing the way to high quality, safety and economy. *N Engl J Med.* 2013;369(17):1581-1583.
15. Kiechle FL, Arcenas RC. Utilization management in a large community hospital. In: Lewandrowski K, ed. *Utilization Management in the Clinical Laboratory and Other Ancillary Services.* New York, NY: Springer; 2017:151-170.

16. Dingle TC, Butler-Wu SM. MALDI-TOF mass spectrometry for microorganism identification. *Clin Lab Med.* 2013;33(3):589-609.
17. Cronin M, Ross JS. Comprehensive next-generation cancer genome sequencing in the era of targeted therapy and personalized oncology. *Biomark Med.* 2011;5(3):293-305.
18. Bianchi DE, Parker L, Wentworth J, et al. DNA sequencing versus standard prenatal aneuploidy screening. *N Engl J Med.* 2014;370(9):799-808.
19. Kiechle FL, Collins L. Clinical laboratory tests not performed in a central hospital laboratory. *J Clin Ligand Assay.* 2005;28(4):198-201.
20. MacMillan D, Lewandrowski E, Lewandrowski K. An analysis of reference laboratory (send out) testing: an 8-year experience in a large academic medical center. *Clin Leadersh Manag Rev.* 2004;18(4):216-219.
21. Worster A. A role for root cause analysis in laboratory medicine. *Lab Med.* 2007;38(12):709-712.
22. Morello RT, Lowthian JA, Barker AL, McGinnes R, Dunt D, Brand C. Strategies for improving patient safety culture in hospitals: a systemwide review. *BMJ Qual Saf.* 2013;22(1):11-18.
23. Kotter JP. *A Sense of Urgency.* Boston, MA: Harvard Business Review Press; 2008.
24. Hicks TE. What ever happened to accountability? *Harvard Business Rev.* 2012; 90(10):93-98.
25. Kiechle FL, Shaw J, Skrisson JE. Outreach implementation requirement: a case study. In: Garcia L, ed. *Clinical Laboratory Management.* 2nd ed. Washington, DC: American Society of Microbiology; 2014:740-759.
26. Howanitz PJ. Errors in laboratory medicine. *Arch Pathol Lab Med.* 2005;129(10):1252-1261.
27. McCay L, Lerner C, Wu AW. Laboratory safety and WHO World Alliance for Patient Safety. *Clin Chim Acta.* 2009;404(1):6-11.
28. Sciacovelli L, Plebani M. The IFCC Working Group on laboratory errors and patient safety. *Clin Chim Acta.* 2009;404(1):79-85.
29. Dasgupta A, Sepulveda JL, eds. *Accurate Results in the Clinical Laboratory: A Guide to Error Detection and Correction.* Amsterdam, Netherlands: Elsevier; 2013.
30. O'Kane M. The reporting, classification and grading of quality failures in the medical laboratory. *Clin Chim Acta.* 2009;404(1):28-31.
31. Carraro C, Plebani M. Errors in a STAT laboratory: types and frequencies 10 years later. *Clin Chem.* 2007;53(7):1338-1342.
32. Plebani M, Carraro P. Mistakes in a stat laboratory: types and frequencies. *Clin Chem.* 1997;43(8):1348-1351.
33. Levick DL, Stern G, Meyerhoefer CO, Pucklavage D. Reducing unnecessary testing in a CPOE system through implementation of a targeted COS intervention. *BMC Med Inform Decis Mak.* 2013;13:43.
34. Huck A, Lewandrowski K. Utilization management in the clinical laboratory: an introduction and overview of the literature. *Clin Chim Acta.* 2014;427(1):111-117.
35. Kiechle FL, Arcenas, RC, Rogers LC. Establishing benchmarks and metrics for disruptive technologies, inappropriate and obsolete tests in the clinical laboratory. *Clin Chim Acta.* 2014;427(1):131-136.
36. Welch WG, Hayes KJ, Frost C. Repeat testing among Medicare beneficiaries. *Arch Intern Med.* 2012;172(22):1745-1751.
37. Kiechle FL, ed. *So You're Going to Collect a Blood Specimen: An Introduction to Phlebotomy.* 15th ed. Northfield, IL: College of American Pathologists; 2017.
38. Korcher DS, Lehman CM. Clinical consequences of specimen rejection: a College of American Pathologists Q-Probes analysis of 78 clinical laboratories. *Arch Pathol Lab Med.* 2014;138(8):1003-1008.
39. Sinici LI, Pinar A, Akbiyik F. Classification of reasons for rejection of biological specimens based on pre-analytical processes to identify quality indicators at a university hospital clinical laboratory in Turkey. *Clin Biochem.* 2014;47(12):1002-1005.
40. Wagar EA, Phipps R, del Guidice R, et al. Inpatient pre-analytic process improvements. *Arch Pathol Lab Med.* 2013;137(12):1753-1760.
41. Valenstein PN, Raab SS, Walsh MK. Identification errors involving clinical laboratories: a College of American Pathologists Q-Probes study of patient and specimen identification errors at 120 institutions. *Arch Pathol Lab Med.* 2006;130(8):1106-1113.
42. Hawker CD, McCarthy W, Cleveland D, Messinger BL. Invention and validation of an automated camera system that uses optical character recognition to identify patient name mislabeled samples. *Clin Chem.* 2014;60(3):463-470.
43. Howanitz PJ, Renner SW, Walsh MK. Continuous wristband monitoring over 2 years decreases identification errors: a College of American Pathologists Q-Tracks study. *Arch Pathol Lab Med.* 2002;126(7):809-815.
44. Phillips SC, Saysona M, Worley S, Hain PD. Reduction in pediatric identification band errors: a quality collaborative. *Pediatrics.* 2012;129(6):e1587-e1593.
45. Glick MR, Ryder KW, Geick SJ, Woods JR. Unreliable visual estimation of the incidence and amount of turbidity, hemolysis and icterus in serum of hospitalized patients. *Clin Chem.* 1989;35(5):837-839.
46. *Hemolysis, Icterus and Lipemia/Turbidity Indices as Indicators of Interference in Clinical Laboratory Analysis. Approved Guideline.* Wayne, PA: Clinical and Laboratory Standards Institute; 2012. Document C56-A.
47. Amukele TK, Sokoll LJ, Pepper D, Howard DP, Street J. Can unmanned aerial systems (drones) be used for the routine transport of chemistry, hematology, and coagulation laboratory specimens? *Plos ONE.* 2015;10(7):e0134020.
48. Keshgegian AA, Bull GE. Evaluation of a soft-handling computerized pneumatic tube specimen delivery system: effects on analytical results and turnaround time. *Am J Clin Pathol.* 1992;97(4):553-540.
49. Shalev V, Chodick G, Heymann AD. Format change of a laboratory test order form affects physician behavior. *Intl J Med Informatics.* 2009;78(10):639-644.
50. Zhi M, Ding EL, Theisen-Toupal J, Whelan J, Arnaout R. The landscape of inappropriate laboratory testing: a 15-year meta-analysis. *Plos ONE.* 2013;8(11):e78962.
51. Jackson BR. Laboratory formularies. *Clin Chim Acta.* 2014;427(1):151-153.

52. Kennedy C, Angermuller S, King R, et al. A comparison of hemolysis rates using intravenous catheter versus venipuncture tubes for obtaining blood samples. *J Emerg Nurs*. 1996;22(6):566-569.
53. Iserson KV. The origins of the gauge system for medical equipment. *J Emerg Med*. 1987;5(1):45-48.
54. *Procedure for the Handling and Processing of Blood Specimens for Common Laboratory Tests. Approved Guideline*. 4th ed. Wayne, PA: Clinical and Laboratory Standards Institute; 2010. Document H18-A4.
55. Howanitz PJ, Lehman CJ, Jones BA, Meier FA, Horowitz GL. Practices for identifying and rejecting hemolyzed specimens are highly variable in clinical laboratories. *Arch Pathol Lab Med*. 2015;139(8):1014-1019.
56. Smith MB. *Sample Quality Assessment for Hemolysis, Icterus and Lipemia/Turbidity*. Technical bulletin for Dimension Vista System. Erlangen, Germany: Siemens; 2013.
57. Nosanchuk JS, Gottmann AW. CUMS and delta checks: a systematic approach to quality control. *Am J Clin Pathol*. 1974;62(5):707-712.
58. Miller I. Development and evaluation of a logical delta check for identifying erroneous blood count results in a tertiary care hospital. *Arch Pathol Lab Med*. 2015;139(8):1042-1047.
59. Sodi R, Darn SM, Stoh A. Pneumatic tube system induced haemolysis: assessing sample type susceptibility to haemolysis. *Ann Clin Biochem*. 2004;41(Pt 3):237-240.
60. Kellerman PS, Thornberrry JM. Pseudohyperkalemia duc to pncumatic tubc transport in a leukemic patient. *Am J Kidney Dis*. 2005;46(4):746-748.
61. Collinson PO, John CM, Gaze DC, Ferrigan LF, Cramp DG. Changes in blood gas samples produced in a pneumatic tube system. *J Clin Pathol*. 2002;55(2):105-107.
62. Da Rin G. Preanalytical workstations: a tool for reducing laboratory errors. *Clin Chim Acta*. 2009;404(1):68-74.
63. Kiechle FL. Workstation consolidation. In: Kiechle FL, Main RI. *The Hitchhiker's Guide to Improving Efficiency in the Clinical Laboratory*. Washington, DC: AACC Press; 2002:45-57.
64. Garm JE. Patient safety and the preanalytic phase of testing. *Clin Leaders Manag Rev*. 2004;18(6):322-327.
65. Stankovic AK, DiLauri E. Quality improvements in the preanalytical phase: focus on urine specimen workflow. *Clin Lab Med*. 2008;28(2):339-350.
66. Aw TC, Kiechle FL. Pseudohyponatremia. *Am J Emerg Med*. 1985;3(3):236-239.
67. Burn J, Gill GV. "Pseudonormonatraemia" *Br Med J*. 1979;2(6198):1110-1111.
68. Fortgens P, Pillay TS. Pseudohyponatremia revisited: a modern-day pitfall. *Arch Pathol Lab Med*. 2011;135(4):516-519.
69. Cybersecurity Vulnerabilities of Hospira Symbiq Infusion System: FDA Safety Communication. US Food and Drug Administration. http://www.fda.gov/MedicalDevices/Safety/AlertsandNotices/ucm456815.htm. July 31, 2015. Updated July 31, 2015. Accessed April 28, 2016.
70. Bonens J, Fokakis M, Armbruster D. Reagent carryover studies: preventing analytical error with open clinical chemistry systems. *Lab Med*. 2005;36(11):705-710.
71. Killeen AA, Long T, Souers R, Ventura CB, Klee GC. Verifying performance characteristics of quantitative analytical systems: calibration verification, linearity, and analytical measurement range. *Arch Pathol Lab Med*. 2014;138(9):1173-1181.
72. Westgard JO, ed. *Basic QC Practices: Training in Statistical Quality Control for Healthcare Laboratories*. 2nd ed. Modian, WI: Westgard QC, Inc; 2002.
73. Sanlidag T, Akcadi S, Ozbakkaloglu B. Serum hepatitis B DNA: stability in relation to multiple freeze-thaw procedures. *J Virol Methods*. 2005;123(1):49-52.
74. Hawker CD, Roberts WI, DaSilva A, et al. Development and validation of an automated thawing and mixing workcell. *Clin Chem*. 2007;53(12):2209-2211.
75. Daves M, Giacomuzzi K, Tagnin E, et al. Influence of centrifuge brake on residual platelet count and routine coagulation tests in citrated plasma. *Blood Coagul Fibrinolysis*. 2014;25(3):292-295.
76. Broughton PMG. Carry-over in automatic analyzers. *J Automatic Chem*. 1984;6(2):94-95.
77. Tate JR, Yen T, Jones GRD. Transference and validation of reference intervals. *Clin Chem*. 2015;61(8):1012-1015.
78. Hawker CD. Laboratory automation: total and subtotal. *Clin Lab Med*. 2007;7(4):749-770.
79. Lippi G, Fostini R, Guidi GC. Quality improvement in laboratory medicine: extra-analytical issues. *Clin Lab Med*. 2008;28(2):285-294.
80. Adeli K, Higgins V, Neeuwesteeg M, et al. Complex reference values for endocrine and special chemistry biomarkers across pediatric, adult and geriatric ages: establishment of robust pediatric and adult reference intervals on the basis of the Canadian Health Measures Survey. *Clin Chem*. 2015;61(8):1063-1074.
81. Adeli K, Raiznman JE, Chen Y, et al. Complex biological profile of hematologic markers across pediatric, adult and geriatric ages: establishment of robust pediatric and adult reference intervals on the basis of the Canadian Health Measures Survey. *Clin Chem*. 2015;61(8):1075-1086.
82. Gardner IH, Safer JD. Progress on the road to better medical care for transgender patients. *Curr Opin Endocrinol Diabetes Obes*. 2013;20(6):553-558.
83. Roberts TK, Kraft CS, French D, et al. Interpreting laboratory results in transgender patients on hormone therapy. *Am J Med*. 2014;127(2):159-162.
84. ECRI Institute. Top 10 health technology hazards for 2014. *Health Devices*. 2013;42(11):1-13.
85. Kiechle FL, Franke DDH. Immunoassays for drugs of abuse: limitations. *J Clin Ligand Assay*. 2007;(3/4):105-112.
86. Snelgrove JW, Jasudavisius AM, Rowe BW, Head EM, Bauer GR. "Completely out-at-sea" with "two-gender medicine": a qualitative analysis of physician-side barriers to providing healthcare for transgender patients. *BMC Health Serv Res*. 2012;12:110.
87. Jones BA, Meier FA. Patient safety in point-of-care testing. *Clin Lab Med*. 2004;24(4):997-1022.
88. Kost GJ. Preventing medical errors in point-of-care testing: security, validation, performance, safeguards and connectivity. *Arch Pathol Lab Med*. 2001;125(10):1307-1315.

89. Kiechle FL, Ingram R, Karcher R, Sykes E. Transfer of glucose measurements outside the laboratory. *Lab Med.* 1990;21(8):504-511.
90. Kiechle FL. Point-of-care testing: one view of past, present and future challenges. *Point of Care.* 2015;14:157-164.
91. Louie RF, Ferguson WJ, Curtis CM, Truong A-T, Lim MH, Kost GJ. The impact of environmental stress on diagnostic testing and implications for patient care during crisis response. In: Kost GJ, Curtis CM, eds. *Global Point of Care: Strategies for Disasters, Emergencies and Public Health Resilience.* Washington, DC: AACC Press; 2015:293-306.
92. Kiechle FL. Point-of-care testing for body fluids. In: Kost GJ, ed. *Principles and Practice of Point-of-Care Testing.* Philadelphia, PA: Lippincott, Williams & Wilkins; 2002: 267-283.
93. Nichols JH. Point-of-care testing. *Clin Lab Med.* 2007;27(4):893-908.
94. Kiechle FL, Gauss I, Robinson-Dunn B. Provider-performed microscopy. *Point of Care.* 2003;2(1):20-32.
95. Kiechle FL, Gauss I. Provider-performed microscopy. *Clin Lab Med.* 2009;29(3):573-582.
96. deVries C, Doggen C, Hibers E, et al. Results of a survey among GP practices on how they manage patient safety aspects to point-of-care testing in every day practice. *BMC Family Pract.* 2015;16:9.
97. Cantero M, Redondo M, Martin E, Callejón G, Hortas ML. Use of quality indicators to compare point-of-care testing errors in a neonatal unit and errors in a STAT central laboratory. *Clin Chem Lab Med.* 2015;53(2):239-247.
98. Ehrmeyer SS. Plan for quality to improve patient safety at the point of care. *Ann Saudi Med.* 2011;31(4):342-346.
99. O'Kane MJ, McManus, P, McGowan N, Lynch PL. Quality error rate in point-of-care testing. *Clin Chem.* 2011;57(9):1267-1271.
100. Baker EH, Wood DM, Brennan AL, Baines DL, Philips BJ. New insights into the glucose oxidase stick test for cerebrospinal fluid rhinorrhoea. *Emerg Med J.* 2005;22(8):556-557.
101. Burstain JM, Brecher ME, Workman K, Foster M, Faber GH, Mair D. Rapid identification of bacterially contaminated platelets using reagent strips: glucose and pH analysis as markers of bacterial metabolism. *Transfusion.* 1997;37(3):255-258.
102. Stormer M, Vollmer T. Diagnostic methods for platelet bacteria screening: current status and developments. *Transfus Med Hemother.* 2014; 41(1):19-27.
103. Martin-Martin C, Martinez-Capoccioni G, Serramito-Garcia R, Espinosa-Restrepo F. Surgical challenge: endoscopic repair of cerebrospinal fluid leak. *BMC Res Notes.* 2012;5:459.
104. Hortensius J, Slingerland RJ, Kleefstra N, et al. Self-monitoring of blood glucose: the case of the first or second drop of blood. *Diabetes Care.* 2011;34(3):556-560.
105. Atkin SH, Dasmaphapatra A, Jaker MA, Chorost MI, Reddy S. Fingerstick glucose determination in shock. *Ann Intern Med.* 1991;114(12):1020-1024.
106. Tonyushkina K, Nichol JH. Glucose meters: a review of technical challenges to obtaining accurate results. *J Diab Sci Technol.* 2009;3(4):971-989.
107. Joseph JI. Analysis: new point-of-care blood glucose monitoring system for hospital demonstrates satisfactory analytical accuracy using blood from critically ill patients: an important step toward improved blood glucose control in the hospital. *J Diab Sci Technol.* 2013;7(5):1288-1293.
108. Alreja G, Setia N, Nichols J, Pantanowitz L. Reducing patient identification errors related to glucose point-of-care testing. *J Pathol Inform.* 2011;2:22.
109. Kanji S, Buffic J, Hutton B, et al. Reliability of point-of-care testing for glucose measurement in critically ill adults. *Crit Care Med.* 2005;33(12):2778-2785.
110. Karon BS, Griesmann L, Scott R, et al. Evaluation of the impact of hematocrit and other interferences in the accuracy of hospital-based glucose meters. *Diabetes Technol Ther.* 2008;10(2):111-120.
111. Tran NR, Godwin ZR, Backhold JC, Passerini AG, Cheng J, Ingemason M. Clinical impact of sample interference in intensive insulin therapy in severely burned patients. *J Burn Care Res.* 2014;35(1):72-79.
112. Finfer S, Wernerman J, Preiser J-C, et al. Clinical review: consensus recommendations on measurement of blood glucose and reporting glycemic control in critically ill adults. *Crit Care.* 2013;17(3):229.
113. Kiechle FL, Main RI. Blood glucose: measurement in the point-of-care setting. *Lab Med.* 2000;31(5):276-282.
114. Karon B. Using glucose meters in intensive care units. *Clin Lab News.* 2015;41(1):28.
115. Li Y, Bai Z, Li M, et al. U-shaped relationship between early blood glucose and mortality in critically ill children. *BMC Pediatrics.* 2015;15:88.
116. Nakhleh RE. Patient safety and error reduction in surgical pathology. *Arch Pathol Lab Med.* 2008;132(2):181-185.
117. Silverman JF. Recent trends in quality, patient safety, and error reduction in nongyn cytology. *Adv Anat Pathol.* 2010;17(6):437-444.
118. Roy JE, Hunt JL. Detection and classification of diagnostic discrepancies (errors) in surgical pathology. *Adv Anat Pathol.* 2010;17(5):359-365.
119. Renshaw AA, Gould EW. Reducing false-negative and false-positive diagnoses in anatomic pathology consultation material. *Arch Pathol Lab Med.* 2013;137(12):1770-1773.
120. Pantanowitz L, Mackinnon AC, Sinard JH. Tracking in anatomic pathology. *Arch Pathol Lab Med.* 2013;137(12):1798-1810.
121. Vollmer RT. Regarding workload and error rates in anatomic pathology. *Am J Clin Pathol.* 2006;126(6):833.
122. Layfield LJ, Anderson GM. Specimen labeling errors in surgical pathology. *Am J Clin Pathol.* 2010;134(3):486-470.
123. Middleton LP, Feeley TW, Albright HW, Walters R, Hamilton SH. Second-opinion pathologic review is a patient safety mechanism that helps reduce errors and decrease waste. *J Oncol Pract.* 2014;10(4):275-280.
124. Kornstein MJ, Byrne SP. The medicolegal aspect of error in pathology: a search of jury verdicts and settlements. *Arch Pathol Lab Med.* 2007;131(4):615-618.

125. Bixenstine PJ, Zarbo RJ, Holzmuller CG, et al. Developing and pilot testing practical measures of pre-analytic surgical specimen identification defects. *Am J Med Qual.* 2013;28(4):308-314.
126. Zarbo RJ, Tuthill M, D'Angelo R, et al. The Henry Ford Production System: reduction of surgical pathology in-process misidentification defects by bar code-specified work process standardization. *Am J Clin Pathol.* 2009;131(4):468-477.
127. Geller BM, Nelson HD, Carney PA, et al. Second opinion in breast pathology: policy, practice and perception. *J Clin Pathol.* 2014;67(11):955-960.
128. Zarbo RJ, Meur FA, Raab SS. Error detection in anatomic pathology. *Arch Pathol Lab Med.* 2005;129(10):1237-1245.
129. Worsham MJ, Wolman SR, Zarbo RJ. Molecular approaches to identification of tissue contamination in surgical pathology sections. *J Mol Diagn.* 2001;3(1):11-15.
130. Gomes DS, Porto SS, Balabram D, Gobbi H. Interobserver variability between general pathologists and a specialist in breast pathology in the diagnosis of lobular neoplasia, columnar cell lesions, atypical ductal hyperplasia and ductal carcinoma in situ of the breast. *Diagn Pathol.* 2014;9:121.
131. Meier FA, Varney RC, Zarbo RJ. Study of amended reports to evaluate and improve surgical pathology processes. *Adv Anat Pathol.* 2011;18(5):406-413.
132. Volmar KE, Idowu MO, Hunt JL, et al. Surgical pathology report defects: a College of American Pathologists Q-Probes study of 73 institutions. *Arch Pathol Lab Med.* 2014;138(5):602-612.
133. Plebani M, Sciacovelli L, Aita A, Chiozza ML. Harmonization of pre-analytical quality indicators. *Biochem Med.* 2014;24(1):105-113.
134. Grecu DS, Vald DC, Duminitrascu V. Quality indicators in the preanalytical phase of testing in a stat laboratory. *Lab Med.* 2014;45(1):74-81.
135. Bachner P. Anniversary of Q-Probes and Q-Tracks quality assurance program. *Arch Pathol Lab Med.* 2014;138(9):1139-1140.
136. Nakhleh RE, Souers RJ, Bashleben CP, et al. Fifteen years' experience of a College of American Pathologists program for continuous monitoring and improvement. *Arch Pathol Lab Med.* 2014;138(9):1150-1155.
137. Meier FA, Souers RJ, Howanitz PJ, et al. Seven Q-tracks monitors of laboratory quality drive general performance improvement: experience from the College of American Pathologists Q-Tracks program 1999-2011. *Arch Pathol Lab Med.* 2015;139(6):762-775.
138. Twarek JA, Volmar KE, McCall SJ, Bashleben CP, Howanitz PJ. Q-Probe studies in anatomic pathology: quality improvement through targeted benchmarking. *Arch Pathol Lab Med.* 2014;138(9):1156-1166.
139. Howanitz PJ, Perrotta PL, Bashleben CP, et al. Twenty-five years of accomplishments of the College of American Pathologists Q-Probes program for clinical pathology. *Arch Pathol Lab Med.* 2014;138(9):1141-1149.
140. Epner PL, Gans JE, Graber ML. When diagnostic testing leads to harm: a new outcomes-based approach for laboratory medicine. *BMJ Qual Saf.* 2013;22:ii6-ii10.
141. *Laboratory Quality Control Based on Risk Management. Approved Guideline.* Wayne, PA: Clinical and Laboratory Standards Institute; 2011. Document EP23-A.
142. Njoroge SW, Nichols JH. Risk management in the clinical laboratory. *Ann Lab Med.* 2014;34(4):274-278.
143. Dintzis SM, Stetsenko GY, Sitlani CM, Gronowski AM, Astion ML, Gallagher TH. Communicating pathology and laboratory errors: anatomic pathologists' and laboratory medical directors' attitudes and experiences. *Am J Clin Pathol.* 2011;135(5):760-765.
144. Gallagher TH, Studdert D, Levinson W. Disclosing harmful medical errors to patients. *N Engl J Med.* 2007;356(26):2713-2719.
145. Pham JC, Girard T, Pronovost PJ. What to do with healthcare incident reporting systems. *J Publ Health Res.* 2013;2:e27.
146. de Feijter JM, de Grave WS, Muijtjens AM, Scherpbier JGA, Koopmans RP. A comprehensive overview of medical error in hospitals using incident-reporting systems, patient complaints and chart review of inpatient deaths. *Plos ONE.* 2012;7(2):e31125.
147. Kohn LT, Corrigan JM, Donaldson MS, eds; Committee on Quality of Health Care in America; Institute of Medicine. *To Err is Human: Building a Safer Health System.* Washington, DC: National Academy Press; 2000.
148. Guillod O. Medical error disclosure and patient safety: legal aspects. *J Publ Health Res.* 2013;2:e31.
149. Nakhleh RE. Disclosure of errors in pathology and laboratory medicine. *Am J Clin Pathol.* 2011;135(5):666-667.
150. Gallagher TH, Mello MM, Levinson W, et al. Talking with patients about other clinicians' errors. *N Engl J Med.* 2013;369(3):1752-1757.
151. Cohen DA, Allen TC, Pathologists and medical error disclosure: don't wait for an invitation. *Arch Pathol Lab Med.* 2015;139(2):163-164.
152. *The Joint Commission Hospital Accreditation Standards, 2001.* Oakbrook Terrace, IL: Joint Commission Resources; 2001.
153. Kachalia A, Kaufman SR, Boothman R, et al. Liability claims and costs before and after implementation of a medical error disclosure program. *Ann Intern Med.* 2010;153(4):213-221.
154. Adams MA, Elmunzer BJ, Scheiman JM. Effect of a health system's medical error disclosure program on gastroenterology-related claims rates and costs. *Am J Gastroenterol.* 2014;109(4):460-464.
155. Bishop A, Fleming M. Patient safety and engagement at the frontlines of healthcare. *Healthcare Qual.* 2014;17(special issue):36-40.
156. Christie A. *Halloween Party.* New York, NY: Harper Collins, 1969.
157. Frankel AS, Leonard MW, Denham CR. Fair and just culture, team behavior, and leadership engagement: the tools to achieve high reliability. *Health Serv Res.* 2006;41(4 Pt 2):1690-1709.
158. Boysen PG. Just culture: a foundation for balanced accountability and patient safety. *Ochsner J.* 2013;13(3):400-406.

3

Human Factors and Patient Safety in the Laboratory

Scott R. Owens, MD

Introduction

Laboratory safety has been under increasing focus since the Clinical Laboratory Improvement Amendments of 1988 (CLIA '88), and the quality of medical care received further attention with the publication of the Institute of Medicine (IOM; now the National Academy of Medicine [NAM]) report, *To Err is Human: Building a Safer Health System*, in 2000.[1] Subsequently, the IOM produced a follow-up document, *Crossing the Quality Chasm: A New Health System for the 21st Century*, which made it clear that improvements in patient safety must not be made at the expense of effective, patient-centered, timely, efficient, and equitable care for all patients.[2] A variety of strides have been made in patient safety and quality health care in the wake of these publications, and clinical laboratories have been leaders in many of these areas. Nonetheless, medicine in general, including laboratory medicine in particular, has not yet achieved the goal of becoming a true "high-reliability organization," despite these efforts.[3] The complexity with which most laboratories operate offers particular difficulties in accomplishing this aim, reflected in the myriad ways in which laboratory testing can go awry, throughout the three phases—preanalytic, analytic, and postanalytic—of specimen (or other patient asset) handling, analysis, and reporting.

As part of the laboratory approach to patient safety and diagnostic accuracy, the study of *human factors and ergonomics* (HFE), sometimes also known as *human factors engineering*, has received increased focus, especially since the publication in 2005 of *Building a Better Delivery System: A New Engineering/Health Care Partnership* by the IOM and the National Academy of Engineering, in which the case was made that attention to systems engineering and health care processes was essential to improving patient safety.[4,5] These human factors include physical, cognitive, and organizational components, covering such diverse issues as the physical layout of a work environment, the "cognitive strain" of a process on the worker, and the effectiveness of teamwork in the organization.[6] Although strides have been made in quality improvement and patient safety in medicine over the last few decades, some observers argue that true and lasting changes in the US health care system cannot be made without additional attention to HFE as related to the complex technological workflow and process inherent in medical practice over the spectrum of professionals involved in patient care.[4,7,8] A reasonable summary view of HFE, vis-à-vis laboratory quality endeavors, might be that whereas traditional quality assurance (QA) and quality improvement (QI) activities focus on process exploration and improvement, HFE focuses on the people in the system and on interactions between them and the systems' components. Furthermore, "human factors" in the context of HFE is not equivalent to "human error."[9] Indeed, true human factors analysis seeks to minimize the opportunity for human error not by additional training and diligence, but by studying and modifying the interactions of the human elements of a system with one another and with each of its other components, thereby making the system as a whole resilient to unforeseen occurrences.

The discipline of laboratory medicine has an undeniably pervasive impact on the care of most patients in a health system. Furthermore, it comprises a wide variety of activities in most centers, from pathologists reading glass slides and generating tissue diagnoses in surgical pathology, to an automated line analyzer for blood samples in the hematology laboratory, to the pre-polymerase chain reaction (PCR) and post-PCR rooms in a molecular diagnostics suite. For each of these sites, workflow and processes can vary significantly, and the analytic phase alone occurs in quite different ways and with different impacts from HFE and other factors. As an example, one could argue that a large and important piece of the analytic phase in surgical pathology occurs within the brain of the pathologist—a place where HFE concerns have an undeniable effect, but where each such factor (as well as the analytic process as a whole) can be difficult to outline and assess definitively. On the other hand, many of the analytic laboratories in clinical pathology operate in a way that is very analogous to a manufacturing facility, where the preanalytic, analytic, and postanalytic phases of work can be relatively easily measured, quantified, scrutinized, and changed, if necessary. Furthermore, the glass slides mentioned in the context of surgical pathology practice are produced in a setting more analogous to the clinical pathology laboratory than the diagnostic space in which they are interpreted, and the tissue represented on them may be subjected to additional studies in an immunohistochemistry or molecular diagnostics laboratory. Thus, HFE issues, although important throughout all aspects of laboratory medicine, can be expected to have quite different impacts and approaches depending on where they are being assessed and altered in the "pathology universe."

In this chapter, an overview of HFE as it relates to health care and specifically to laboratory medicine will be outlined. Attention will be placed on the following areas: the roles of manual versus automated tasks; the parts played by equipment design and failures, systems failures, and environmental failures, all as they relate to HFE; the potential impact of HFE-focused systems improvements on error reduction in the laboratory; and the roles of personnel fatigue, stress, scheduling, communication, and teamwork as they relate to laboratory errors.

Human Factors and Ergonomics: A Health Care Perspective

While "systems thinking" and attendant tools—such as the Toyota Production System (TPS), Lean thinking, Total Quality Management (TQM), and others—are increasingly applied to health care (including clinical laboratories), the complex nature of patient care and health care organizations continues to make this approach challenging.[10] The application of HFE principles to the field of patient care also faces the challenges created by this complexity, and the employment of any ergonomic or human factors solution or countermeasure that does not take into account the entire system of the laboratory is unlikely to yield effective or lasting change with regard to the targeted issue, be it patient safety, laboratory errors, or diagnostic accuracy.[7] In addition, a given health care system and its laboratories have both internal and external components and drivers.[7] Internal parts of the system include the physical environment itself (infrastructure, space, etc), the specific health care organization and its characteristics (eg, free-standing community hospital, regional health care system, large national corporation, or public university–based system), and the tools provided and acquired for the system's function (such as a laboratory information system [LIS], electronic health record [EHR], and equipment in the laboratory). External parts of the system include regulatory standards and legislation (such as CLIA), accreditation organizations, and the workforce from which the laboratory's personnel are obtained, which can have significant local variability.

Carayon and others have done much work in applying and studying HFE principles in health care systems broadly.[4,6,7] Some of this work has focused on the so-called SEIPS (Systems Engineering Initiative for Patient Safety) model for health care. This model places the health care delivery enterprise into an overall *work system* that takes into account the internal and external environments and other factors inherent to the system. The specific work *process* for a system (and, by extension, a specific laboratory) is an outgrowth of this work system and its inherent characteristics. This specific process is the target of study for some of the tools referred to earlier (eg, TPS; Lean Thinking), and the effects of the broader work system must be taken into account when using such tools to study and affect processes if the resultant information and changes created by their output are to be effective. Finally, the *outcomes* of the work done by the system and its process(es) are the visible manifestations of its activity. In the context of a laboratory, this can range from the daily output of a chemistry analyzer to the overall clinical outcome for a given patient who receives a tissue diagnosis from a pathologist. Increasingly, the measure of quality for these outputs is shifting from volume to value, and one can reasonably expect that the practice of laboratory medicine will not be exempt from some form of population outcomes–based reimbursement in the future.[11]

As applied to health care, the five components of the work system are (1) the person, (2) the tasks performed, (3) the tools and technology available, (4) the physical environment, and (5) the organization.[7] Put another way, Lowe[12] describes these elements as the "6Ps": providers, procedures, products, peripherals, patients, and policy. While there is increasing information on the effects of these components in the health care system, much of the literature focuses on the activities involved in direct, face-to-face patient care, such as in the operating room or the intensive care unit. In the remainder of this section, each of these five components will be described briefly and placed into the specific context of laboratory medicine.

As outlined by Carayon et al,[7] the *person* is defined as the individual at the center of the system—the one doing the work. Although this terminology implies a single individual, the person can, in fact, be a team of individuals performing the same work. A laboratory-centered example of this might be the team of pathology assistants in a laboratory, who may be focused on gross examinations and sampling of surgical specimens. In addition, depending on the perspective of the system, the "person" at the center may be the patient or a patient group, such as those undergoing hemoglobin A1C measurements in a chemistry laboratory or those waiting for anatomic pathology reports to appear in the patient portal. The person (or team) has unique characteristics that have myriad effects on the system, including physical, cognitive, and emotional characteristics that can affect such wide-ranging aspects as the ability to tolerate a single physical position at a microscope, the degree of training needed for installation of new equipment, or the responses of a laboratory technologist to questions from an inspection team representing an accrediting agency. From the standpoint of the patient, emotional and psychosocial characteristics may have an effect on his or her ability and desire to wait for the result of a tissue biopsy or a molecular diagnostics study.

The *tasks* of a work system are varied and depend on the specific purpose the system serves. With regard to a laboratory, these can include specific and laboratory-centric work such as plating and reading results of microbial cultures, loading a production line–type blood analyzer, or embedding tissue and cutting tissue sections on a microtome. Each of these tasks carries with it a unique set of ancillary characteristics, both physical and psychological. These can include the physical demands of moving equipment and supplies, the psychological demands of keeping up with a busy surgical pathology specimen load, and the need for interpersonal communication as specimens move from one part of the laboratory to another and/or other members of the care team call regarding results. In addition to these patient care–focused tasks, work systems contain a number of other non–care-related (or indirectly related) duties, such as personnel management, physical care for equipment and the environment, and quality assurance activities.

Tools and technology in clinical laboratories are myriad. For example, the degree of complexity in an automated analysis line for hematology assays rivals any other piece of extremely high-technology equipment and can include lasers, robotics, and other entities only dreamt of a few decades ago. In this example, this complexity must be managed by hematology laboratory personnel in addition to their tasks of preparing and reading blood smears with a microscope, preparing bone marrow aspirates and examinations, and, in some cases, examining other body fluids, all using different types of technology and different tools. Analogous tools are part of all other pathology laboratories, and, in addition to these issues, a major part of the work system in any laboratory revolves around use of information technology in the form of the LIS for managing specimen flow and for reporting results. Finally, most hospital laboratories interface their LIS and their operations with the institutional EHR, meaning that laboratory workers must manage this additional level of technology and its inherent benefits and challenges.

The *physical environment* plays a critical role in laboratory function, from the individual benches and workstations for laboratory personnel to the way the laboratory is situated in the hospital or other locale. In many cases, critical functions such as frozen-section laboratories can be "shoehorned" into spaces that are either insufficient to begin with or quickly outgrown because of increased work volume. In the complex ecosystem of a health care system, laboratory functions are often added to facilities that were not originally designed to house them (eg, surgical pathology services added to an outpatient surgery center or point-of-care testing moved into a repurposed room near an intensive care unit). Furthermore, each of these laboratory locations competes for space with the equally important clinical functions of other units, and many pathology departments have separate spaces throughout a health system, raising challenges created by geographic separation. The physical qualities of the facility itself must also be considered; ventilation, temperature control, noise, and other factors have minute-to-minute effects on laboratory workers.

The *organization* in which a laboratory functions has both tangible and intangible effects on the work system. Certainly, a laboratory has a formal organizational structure within which it must function, from departmental to institutional to governmental and regulatory levels. Equally important, however, is the informal structure or culture of a work system. This can have wide-ranging effects on worker productivity and satisfaction, as well as on quality of care and safety of patients. A laboratory functioning in an organizational culture in which challenges posed by any of the other elements of the work system are not met with a team-focused and rational approach is likely to be populated by technologists and other caregivers who feel disconnected from the organization and frustrated with their teammates and their leadership. Specific examples include flimsy support for the LIS or a culture in which hierarchy is emphasized at the expense of practicality, either of which would interfere with effective organizational function and patient care.

Clearly, the myriad interconnections outlined in the paragraphs above suggest that work systems can have complex effects on workers and vice versa. Changes or challenges in one area can have ramifications in one or more of the other areas, with cumulative or even synergistic results. For example, the installation of a new LIS (tools and technologies) is associated with many inherent challenges to workflow in a laboratory system; if departmental or institutional support, either monetary or personnel related, is insufficient to cope with these challenges in a timely fashion (organization), the impact on patient care activities and worker engagement could be significant. Furthermore, insufficient laboratory space (physical environment) can result not only in spatial crowding of workers and equipment, but it may incite ergonomic difficulties for individual workers (person) forced into awkward postures or physical separation of equipment, resulting in inefficient and tiresome workflow (tasks). Although HFE and a systems approach to health care safety have been used to study many such interactions and their effects on the health care system as a whole, there is evidence that these studies have, by-and-large, not yet effectively detailed or recognized the complexity of the connections.[13]

The Role of Automation in the Laboratory

The concept of automation of tasks in the laboratory rose to prominence in the 1990s in the United States, although there was movement in this direction earlier in Japan.[14] To some extent, this trend reflects similar changes in realms outside medicine, such as manufacturing. In all cases, inside and outside the laboratory, the drive toward automation reflects certain motivating forces. These include such things as a shortage of qualified workers, a drive for faster production (in the case of the laboratory, decreased turnaround time), mitigation of increased work volume, and, important in the context of this chapter, an attempt to reduce human errors. This last force can be viewed more broadly in the context of the work system components described in the previous section. In other words, while often serving to decrease the risk of errors introduced by the human components of a work system, laboratory automation also has impacts on and is affected by each of the categories in the context of HFE. As an example, a large automation line in a clinical hematology laboratory must have adequate space (physical environment), adequate technological support and integration into departmental and institutional information technology systems (tools and technology), and accessible and comfortable access for technologists (person).

Laboratory automation can have a variety of forms. *Total automation* implies automated handling of all phases of a specimen's processing, from preanalytic through analytic and postanalytic (results reporting) phases. In this scenario, a worker loads specimens onto an automated analysis line, which carries out the rest of the process through the act of reporting the result, which usually passes directly into the LIS and/or EHR. Afterward, a human worker typically reenters the process to remove any residual specimen for archiving, although some systems have a provision for this portion of the process as well. In this case, only two places remain subject to human error: the sorting and loading of sample, and the storage/archiving phase. Clearly, some laboratory processes are more amenable to this type of automation than others, with clinical chemistry and hematology being the leaders. The work systems in microbiology, molecular diagnostics, and other departments remain too complex for total automation, as do most aspects of anatomic pathology specimen handling.

Another form of automated laboratory function is *modular automation*, which replaces only part(s) of the process. Several different modules can be combined to complete different functions, but human intervention is usually needed to move specimens from one module to the next. Examples might include a specimen-sorting module for the preanalytic phase, coupled with a chemistry module that handles certain analytes, and a hematology module that assesses blood indices; human workers would intervene to move specimen tubes from one freestanding module to the next. This type of system may be more appropriate in the context of certain anatomic pathology functions. An example of this may include an automated embedding and paraffin block–cutting station, which does not entirely omit interaction and manipulation by human histotechnologists but automates a critical part of the process.

Other laboratory functions may be automated, including quality control, inventory, and data reporting (sometimes known as *autoverification*). Each of these types of automation can have benefits to many components of the work system, including laboratory technologists and patients, by reducing turnaround times, laboratory errors, and fatigue induced by repetitive tasks. Nonetheless, laboratory automation, in whatever form it takes, is not a panacea for issues of HFE. Introduction of an automated analysis line can have ramifications for other parts of the laboratory process that may not be initially apparent and that may require additional work to mitigate. For example, certain labels for patient assets such as test tubes may not be compatible with the robotics of an analyzer that move specimens from one phase to the next, resulting in jamming or ejection of tubes from the machine. In addition, computer servers running line analyzers can malfunction, requiring robust manual backup techniques that are quickly executable to ensure that analyses and reporting continues during downtime for the machinery.

Arguably, most of the investigations of the impact of automation in the pathology laboratory setting have been in the blood bank. South et al[15] reported a marked potential decrease in errors in pretransfusion testing when automated "type and screen" (ie, blood group testing and antibody screening) methods were utilized, with evidence provided using failure mode and effects analysis (FMEA). This study indicated as much as a 98% reduction in the opportunity for defects as compared with manual methods of testing, partially due to a marked decrease in the number of process steps between the two approaches. A similar finding with regard to blood bank automation was reported by Han et al,[16] although their primary goal was to study the utility of FMEA itself as a useful tool for laboratory process improvement.

Technology, System, and Process Issues

Clearly, human interaction with patient assets in the laboratory gives opportunities for the introduction of human error that can be mitigated to a large extent by the tools of automated handling of specimens and results. Nonetheless, the steps performed by human beings in the laboratory are only one part of the complex work system, as discussed in the section, "Human Factors and Ergonomics: A Health Care Perspective," above. Indeed, although one method of preventing human error can be the institution of technological solutions, the introduction of technology anywhere in the patient care system, inside or outside the laboratory, can lead to significant patient harm if it does not incorporate both adequate design of the equipment and appropriate instruction of health care workers. For example, although not focused on laboratory equipment, a study of defects and malfunction in surgical instruments indicated that 6% of defective instruments were discovered only in the course of their use (ie, in the operating theater *during* a surgical procedure), creating "near-miss" clinical scenarios with the potential for patient harm.[17]

Many potentially harmful components of the laboratory work system, as well as potentially deleterious interactions between system components, seem to "hide in plain sight."[12,18] That is, they lie in a latent state as "accidents waiting to happen," until the right mixture of conditions and people come together to make an adverse event inevitable. This is why relying on a safety record that simply catalogs days between accidents is never as helpful as a safety system that seeks out potential danger areas and stress-tests the system in anticipation of mishaps. Taking a step further back, issues of device and technology design become critical in preventing the possibility of accidents, at least to some degree.

Often, design is equated with the simple look or feel of a device or of the interface between a device and its intended user. HFE, however, recognizes that a device's design, especially in the setting of health care, should take into account issues of usability and customer (user) feedback in order to ensure a functional and safe design over and above a product that is simply well engineered.[18,19] As outlined by Lowe,[12] there are five elements of device and technology design that are essential for health care applications: usability, reliability, accident-proofing, standardization, and awareness of how the device interacts with the system as a whole. These individual guidelines of design may seem intuitive, but there are numerous reported examples of real and potential patient harm in which these guidelines were not followed or were not optimized. Many of these examples occur in the sphere of direct patient care, such as in the emergency or operating rooms or in medication delivery. There are few examples centered specifically on laboratory testing; nonetheless, parallels can be drawn from some of these reports to processes involving similar principles that are part of laboratory operations. For example, lack of standardization in the user interface and operational characteristics of cardiac defibrillators have led to inadvertent delivery of inappropriate electrical shocks to patients suffering from cardiac arrhythmias (eg, defibrillation doses given instead of synchronized cardioversions).[20] Similarly, variance analysis studies have assessed the opportunities for error that remain despite the institution of a barcode-assisted medication delivery system.[21] There is no reason to think that laboratory devices (or workers) are immune to similar issues, because analyzers and other equipment have complex and nonstandardized user interfaces, and barcode-driven workflow is becoming common in pathology laboratories.

It should be obvious from this discussion that design of the tools and technologies in a work system are of paramount importance to ensuring safe operation and patient care. In order to identify design flaws that potentially undermine these goals, user and usability testing—especially before implementation of new technologies—is highly valuable.[18] Furthermore, customization of interfaces to better fit local systems and workflow as well as a movement toward *graphical user interfaces* for complex technology (versus buttons, dials, etc) have been shown to be beneficial in promoting quality and patient safety.[22] In addition, and especially important for technologies already in use, a robust and open policy fostering reporting of equipment problems is crucial.[19] Not only should this type of policy promote a focus on systems thinking and identification of systematic problems rather than blaming the individual worker, it should also recognize that countermeasures focused on retraining, vigilance, and checklists are no substitute for effective design principles and a focus on error-proofing laboratory operations (ie, focusing on device and workflow design that makes it *more difficult to fail* than to perform within expectations). Some approaches to error-proofing include the use of appropriate checklists to maintain the order and integrity of complex processes and the use of "forcing functions" (often involving computerized workflow) to ensure that crucial steps in the process are not omitted. It must be recognized, however, that such countermeasures need to be balanced with other aspects of the work system (such as time, workload, and competing priorities) in order to avoid the creation of potential workarounds that further compromise the system in the misguided interest of increasing perceived efficiency.

Clearly, the design of medical devices and technologies is critical to how they function and, particularly from the standpoint of HFE principles, how the person (usually people) in the system interacts with them. Just as important, however, is the physical design of the environment itself. No amount of machine design can substitute for a well-planned and well-laid out workspace, and the physical layout of spaces has both physical and mental impacts on the workers utilizing them, particularly in the complex work system of health care in general and in the laboratory in particular.

One way to maximize the utility and workability of a space is to create "spaghetti diagrams" of the work being done there.[23] This tool, often used in the context of Lean principles, uses a scale drawing of the space, over which are laid lines representing the physical movements of workers in the space as they go about their jobs (Figure 3-1). By doing this exercise in the "before" (or current) state, followed by changes in the physical layout of the space and repeated mapping exercises, a more efficient physical workflow can be obtained, maximizing worker time and minimizing excess movement and energy expenditure. Exercises such as this can sometimes result in manifold increases in efficiency and equally impressive decreases in time expenditure, leaving more time for other activities by highly skilled staff. A concrete example might be in a molecular diagnostics laboratory, where several separate spaces (eg, pre-PCR and post-PCR areas) may be necessary for proper specimen handling. Appropriate proximity of these spaces with an optimized physical workflow and placement of equipment means not only increased worker productivity and satisfaction but also potentially fewer specimen contaminations and errors. Similar exercises can be used in the context of specimen transport and information workflow in an LIS.

Other potential environmental and systems issues may be more or less within the control of the laboratory personnel and leadership, although they must still be in the overall calculation of factors affecting the system as a whole. For example, delicate laboratory and computer equipment may be rendered

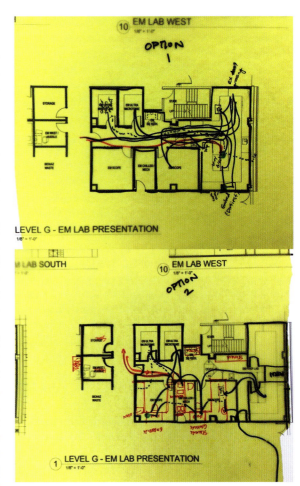

Figure 3-1. Example of a "spaghetti diagram" used in space and ergonomic planning. The space layout shown in option 2 (bottom panel) was estimated to create a 48% more efficient use of technologist movement (based on total feet walked) versus the layout in option 1 (top panel). These comparative diagrams were created during a 30-minute session involving technologists who were going to be using the proposed space. (Images courtesy of Corrie Pennington-Block and Laurie DaForno.)

functionless (or put into protective standby mode) by vibrations from heavy equipment working in a nearby parking lot or other construction project. Hospital projects involving interruption of water flow or electricity may make contingency plans necessary, such as backup generators, to maintain continuous service in the laboratory. Temperature-monitoring systems can be useful in protecting equipment and specimens at appropriate operating and/or preservation temperatures. The point of these examples is not to create a laundry list of responsibilities and potential pitfalls for the laboratory manager reading this chapter, but to point out the myriad ways that elements of the laboratory system as a whole—including laboratory technologists and patients—interact and affect each other.

Teams, Fatigue, Stress, and Scheduling

As discussed thus far in this chapter, HFE principles emphasize the often complex interaction of all parts of the work system specifically as they relate to actions by and effects on the human components (person) of the system. Although the term *person* is used to connote these human members of the system, in many cases we have seen that more than one person is involved. Furthermore, in the context of health care, this human element can be on either the caregiving side or on the receiving side (patient) of the system. Particularly on the side of caregiving in the high-value and high-stakes world of health care, issues of teamwork, person-to-person interactions, stress, and fatigue become important components of the overall system and its function.

Some aspects of these interpersonal, cognitive, and social interactions between team members have been termed *nontechnical skills*, which complement the many technical and diagnostic skills of laboratory team members.[24] These skills have been categorized as *situational awareness, decision making, communication, teamwork, leadership, stress management,* and *coping with fatigue*; as with technical skills, in many cases nontechnical skills can be learned, suggesting that emphasis on such abilities in training laboratory personnel may be useful in optimizing the human factors of the complex laboratory work system. The ways in which these skills can affect laboratory function and patient safety are numerous, but a few specific examples include specimen (patient) handoffs; communication of laboratory and diagnostic errors among team members and to patients; recognition of situations potentially impairing one's judgment and cognition, such as a challenging frozen section diagnosis, a higher-than-usual daily workload, time pressure caused by urgent inquiries about results on a critical patient, and so forth.

Much of what we know about the functions of teams in the health care setting comes from recognized high-risk situations involving multiple team members, such as in the operating room, and is reported in the literature in anesthesiology and surgery.[25] In turn, much of this knowledge comes by way of strides made a number of decades ago in other high-risk (and, ultimately, high-reliability) settings, such as in the aviation industry and space flight programs. Lewis et al[25] presented a series of concepts from the aviation industry with direct applications to health care in a 2011 report in *The Milbank Quarterly*. The crux of this report suggests several potential initiatives in the health care sphere that stem from HFE principles, but perhaps the most compelling assertion is that one concept, "counterheroism," can be of paramount importance.

The history of the commercial aviation industry for most of the 20th century involved a pilot whose word, in the cockpit, was irrefutable. After a number of examples of airline disasters stemming from human error, compounded by a "cockpit culture" in which other team members' observations and judgments were subservient to those of the pilot, much study and HFE work contributed to a series of changes that put more autonomy and responsibility in the hands of other members of the flight crew. Some of this work culminated in a system of crew resource management (CRM) training, in which the importance of all available resources (people, equipment, and information) in the conduct of flight is emphasized. This concept has been translated to medicine in such environments as the operating room, where CRM-inspired and other aviation-inspired countermeasures such as checklists and time-outs continue to struggle somewhat against the heroism culture still ingrained in medicine. In this culture, workarounds and non–systems-based solutions to problems—such as changes in intraoperative (or laboratory) protocol that involve nonstandard use of tools and technology or other "on-the-fly" strategies to counter unanticipated events in patient care—are celebrated, whereas a systems approach to problem solving is seen as compromising or questioning the judgment and ability of the practitioner.[25] As a specific example, the hero culture in laboratory medicine might put a premium on a practitioner who could make a difficult diagnosis on poorly cut frozen section slides with a high level of demand from a surgeon for an accurate intraoperative diagnosis in a VIP patient. The systems-based culture, on the other hand, would ask why the processing system for frozen section slides resulted in poorly cut slides in the first place and, further, why the process should run differently for any one patient, VIP or not. There is evidence that CRM training provides a highly positive return on investment in the setting of medicine.[26]

A systems-based and protocol-based operation structure can be thought of as a "counterheroism" approach to medical practice, a methodology that has resulted in amazing advances in safety over the past several decades in the commercial aviation industry when utilized not only by cockpit crew but by mechanics, cabin crew, and others.[25] Although this type of protocol-driven operation can be thought of as incorporating such tools as checklists and electronic procedures, it is not limited to those countermeasures. Rather, it involves a much broader modification of behaviors and approaches to activities—such as fostering a culture in which any member of the laboratory team can raise concerns about a process or decision—and creating a safe space to encourage self-reporting of errors, near-misses, and concerns in an attempt to learn from every real or potential error. These tenets can be extended to other important aspects of team and individual workflow, including stress reduction; management activities and coaching; recognition of fatigue and its effects; and a scheduling, staffing and workload distribution approach that works toward these ends as well.

Some observers have argued that the systems approach to health care that is advocated by HFE principles may result in an abrogation of personal responsibility for safety in the laboratory and elsewhere in the health care system.[27,28] There is evidence, however, that this is not the case. Indeed, a "just culture" approach to identifying and mitigating medical errors has proven to be an effective way of fostering the type of culture that raises real and potential errors to the level of recognition that each such event is a chance for the system to learn a lesson and improve. Although willful misconduct and gross negligence should be identified and rooted out of the system in the name of safety and reliability, blaming the operator for errors and relying on diligence and conscientiousness to prevent them are not constructive or effective measures and should be eradicated with a careful, systems-based identification of root causes and potential countermeasures.

Summary

Quality assurance, quality improvement, and patient safety have been a focus of medical practice and research for nearly two decades. The practice of laboratory medicine has incorporated many quality control metrics and practices in its daily work for much longer than that; however, much work remains to be done in the realm of quality improvement and, specifically, in the arena of human factors and ergonomics as it relates to the many aspects of pathology practice, including the clinical laboratories and anatomic pathology. Systems-based thinking and analysis of the entirety of complex interactions of all aspects of a laboratory work system (person, tasks, tools and technology, physical environment, and organization) is central to the concept of HFE and provides useful tools to increase safety and value for all members of the health care equation, both providers and patients.

References

1. Kohn LT, Corrigan JM, Donaldson MS, eds; Committee on Quality of Health Care in America; Institute of Medicine. *To Err is Human: Building a Safer Health System.* Washington, DC: National Academy Press; 2000.
2. Richardson WC, Berwick DM, Bisgard JC, eds; Committee on Quality of Health Care in America; Institute of Medicine. *Crossing the Quality Chasm: A New Health System for the 21st Century.* Washington, DC: National Academy Press; 2001.
3. Sutcliffe K. High reliability organizations (HROs). *Best Pract Res Clin Anaesthesiol.* 2011;25:133-144.
4. Hignett S, Carayon P, Buckle P, Catchpole K. State of science: human factors and ergonomics in healthcare. *Ergonomics.* 2013;56:1491-1503.
5. Reid PP, Compton WD, Grossman JH, Fanjiang G, eds. *Building a Better Delivery System: A New Engineering/Health Care Partnership.* Washington, DC: National Academies Press; 2005.
6. Xie A, Carayon P. A systematic review of human factors and ergonomics (HFE)-based healthcare system redesign for quality of care and patient safety. *Ergonomics.* 2015;58:33-49.
7. Carayon P, Wetterneck TB, Rivera-Rodriguez AJ, et al. Human factors systems approach to healthcare quality and patient safety. *Appl Ergon.* 2014;45:14-25.
8. Buckle P, Clarkson PJ, Coleman R, Ward J, Anderson J. Patient safety, systems design and ergonomics. *Appl Ergon.* 2006;37:491-500.
9. Russ AL, Fairbanks RJ, Karsh B-T, Militello LG, Saleem JJ, Wears RL. The science of human factors: separating fact from fiction. *BMJ Qual Saf.* 2013;22:802-808.
10. Hignett S, Jones EL, Miller D, et al. Human factors and ergonomics and quality improvement science: integrating approaches for safety in healthcare. *BMJ Qual Saf.* 2015;24:250-254.
11. Schmidt RL, Ashwood ER. Laboratory medicine and value-based health care. *Am J Clin Pathol.* 2015;144:357-358.
12. Lowe CM. Accidents waiting to happen: the contribution of latent conditions to patient safety. *Qual Saf Health Care.* 2006;15(Suppl 1):i72-i75.
13. Waterson P. A critical review of the systems approach within patient safety research. *Ergonomics.* 2009;52:1185-1195.
14. Rodriques, S. Guidelines for implementing automation in a hospital laboratory setting, part I. *Clin Leadersh Manag Rev.* 2007;21:E2.
15. South SF, Casina TS, Li L. Exponential error reduction in pretransfusion testing with automation. *Transfusion.* 2012;52:81S-87S.
16. Han TH, Kim MJ, Kim S, et al. The role of failure modes and effects analysis in showing the benefits of automation in the blood bank. *Transfusion.* 2013;53:1077-1082.
17. Yasuhara H, Fukatsu K, Komatsu T, Obayashi T, Saito Y, Uetera Y. Prevention of medical accidents caused by defective surgical instruments. *Surgery.* 2012;151:153-161.

18. Gosbee JW. Conclusion: You need human factors engineering expertise to see design hazards that are hiding in "plain sight!" *Jt Comm J Qual Saf.* 2004;30:696-700.
19. Newton RC, Mytton OT, Aggarwal R, et al. Making existing technology safer in healthcare. *Qual Saf Health Care.* 2010;19(Suppl 2):i15-i24.
20. Fairbanks RJ, Caplan S. Poor interface design and lack of usability testing facilitate medical error. *Jt Comm J Qual Saf.* 2004;30:579-584.
21. Escoto KH, Hallock M, Wagner J, Karsh B-T. Using variance analysis to detect hazards in a bar-code–assisted medication preparation process. *Jt Comm J Qual Saf.* 2004;30:622-628.
22. Burkolter D, Weyers B, Kluge A, Luther W. Customization of user interfaces to reduce errors and enhance user acceptance. *Appl Ergon.* 2014;45:346-353.
23. Skeldon SC, Simmons A, Hersey K, et al. Lean methodology improves efficiency in outpatient academic uro-oncology clinics. *Urology.* 2014;83:992-997.
24. Johnston PW, Fioratou E, Flin R. Non-technical skills in histopathology: definition and discussion. *Histopathology.* 2011;59:359-367.
25. Lewis GH, Vaithianathan R, Hockey PM, Hirst G, Bagian JP. Counterheroism, common knowledge, and ergonomics: concepts from aviation that could improve patient safety. *Milbank Q.* 2011;89:4-38.
26. Moffatt-Bruce SD, Hefner JL, Mekhjian H, et al. What is the return on investment for implementation of a crew resource management program at an academic medical center? *Am J Med Qual.* 2015;31:1-7.
27. Dekker SWA, Leveson NG. The systems approach to medicine: controversy and misconceptions. *BMJ Qual Saf.* 2015;24:7-9.
28. Amalberti R, Auroy Y, Berwick D, et al. Five system barriers to achieving ultrasafe healthcare. *Ann Intern Med.* 2005;142:756-764.

4

Communication, Handoffs, and Transitions

Virginia Elizabeth Duncan, MD
Suzanne Renée Thibodeaux, MD, PhD
Gene P. Siegal, MD, PhD

Communication in Anatomic and Clinical Pathology Laboratories

The term *patient safety* has become a recent buzzword in medicine, although the concept has been around since before Hippocrates. The idea of systematized error prevention came sometime later, but in modern times it was brought conspicuously into the international spotlight with the publication of the 2000 Institute of Medicine report, *To Err Is Human*,[1] and their 2001 follow-up report, *Crossing the Quality Chasm*.[2] (See also their 2015 addition to the series, *Improving Diagnosis in Health Care*.[3]) Since the initial 2000 report, we have seen an explosion of patient safety initiatives in all specialties of medicine.

In pathology and laboratory medicine, there is a long tradition of structured strategies for generating and managing accurate and clinically relevant information. For decades, clinical and anatomic pathology laboratories have had systems-based processes in place for monitoring and maintaining the quality of each test or procedure. *Quality* is our patient safety measure, which can be broadly conceptualized as error prevention combined with improvement of care. *Quality control* refers to quality-maintaining systems at the level of each individual test or procedure, and *quality assurance* is the umbrella that encompasses and integrates the individual quality control systems. These systems are subjected to rigorous and repetitive oversight, measures of performance, and, in many cases, retrospective review.[4] This ongoing and continually evolving process continues to be extensively studied, and the literature is rich with examples of quality management analysis and available tools to prevent errors and improve laboratory information output (for example, College of American Pathologists [CAP] Q-Probes and Q-Tracks[5]).

Less well studied is the importance of communication in the laboratory. Studies that do exist tend to focus on the communication of critical laboratory values or the communication of diagnoses between pathologist and clinician, particularly with respect to the details of the official pathology report[6-8] (also see the discussion in the next section). Pathology is a consultative service, and this type of communication is critical, but the story is more complicated than that. A complex chain of information transfers occurs, beginning when the patient undergoes his or her procedure or specimen collection and ending when the results of diagnostic testing are communicated (usually via the clinician) back to the patient (or to the patient's family in the case of a child, a mentally incompetent adult, or an autopsy). With any break in that chain, information may be lost and patient safety can be compromised.

In the anatomic and clinical pathology laboratories, this information chain can be divided into three phases of testing: the preanalytic phase, in which specimens are prepared for testing; the analytic phase, which comprises the actual diagnostic procedures; and the postanalytic phase, in which the results of the tests are generated and communicated. Most laboratory-related medical errors (and thus much of the potential harm to patients) occur in the preanalytic and postanalytic phases.[9]

In the preanalytic phase, before testing occurs, specimens pass through many hands on their way from patient to pathologist. Collection, labeling, and transport occur before arrival in the laboratory, and pretest intralaboratory accessioning, transport, and processing follow. Errors in this phase are typically due to specimen mislabeling or mishandling, issues common to both anatomic and clinical pathology. A CAP Q-Probes investigation of the mislabeling and wrong-blood-in-tube (WBIT) error rates at blood banks of 122 institutions found a mislabeled sample rate of 1.12% and WBIT rate of 0.04%.[10] Although patient outcomes were not specifically studied, these findings highlight the potential for significant morbidity when, for example, ABO incompatibility complicates these errors. On the surgical pathology side, a recent CAP Q-Probes study of 136 institutions found an overall mislabeling rate of 0.4%. Of these, 1.3% of cases were judged to have affected patient care. Most errors, however, were caught and corrected in the course of specimen processing.[11]

With the rise of personalized medicine and prognostic/therapeutic biomarkers, a new and rapidly expanded cadre of potential errors is arising. One example is the requirement to fix specimens for specific periods of time to maximize consistency and reproducibility (estrogen receptor/progesterone receptor determination for breast cancer being the best-known recent example). Thus, one must now track and document tissue from intraoperative vascular clamping to accessioning in the laboratory and during placement in the appropriate fixative from a specific start to stop time.[12] Systems-based interventions such as computerized routing and scanning technology can mitigate—but not completely abrogate—many specimen-handling errors and are increasingly being implemented.

Critical Values Reporting

In the postanalytic phase of testing, the reporting of critical values is one of the better-studied and potentially important types of communication in the laboratory. Lundberg[13] first defined the concept of critical values in 1972 as a laboratory test result that could indicate a life-threatening emergency. Since then, reporting of critical values has become widespread in laboratories and mandated by accrediting agencies worldwide. Historically, the concept was limited to the clinical laboratory, but in recent years many authors have advocated broadening it to include anatomic pathology as well.

The Joint Commission (formerly the Joint Commission on Accreditation of Healthcare Organizations [JCAHO]) states in its National Patient Safety Goal 2: "Improve the effectiveness of communication among caregivers," with one of its specific requirements to "develop ... [and] implement the procedures for managing the critical results of tests and diagnostic procedures."[14] Whereas the application to laboratory medicine is obvious, surgical pathology and cytopathology could be assumed to fall under the rubric of "diagnostic procedures."

The Clinical Laboratory Improvement Amendments of 1988 (CLIA '88) treats the issue more generally, without distinguishing between anatomic and clinical pathology. Two of its standards for laboratory accreditation are "Communication" and "Test Report," stating that laboratories must have in place systems to (1) identify breakdowns in communication and (2) ensure accurate, timely, and reliable transfer of data from laboratory to clinician.[15] Critical values can be assumed to fall within the category of communication in general.

The CAP Laboratory Accreditation Program (LAP) casts a wider net, defining "significant and unexpected ... findings," rather than "critical values." It includes within its checklist examples of possible significant, unexpected findings pertaining to anatomic pathology with a statement that the specifics are to be determined by the individual pathology department.[6] Specific requirements for reporting are not currently mandated by any accrediting agency, and reporting systems tend to be heterogeneous.

Recommendations and general guidelines do exist, particularly for the clinical laboratory. For example, in 2010 Singh et al[16] published recommendations for institutions seeking to craft or revise critical values reporting policies. Choices of which tests to report and at what thresholds are laboratory specific and particularly variable, although attempts at standardization have been made. This has led many to question whether greater consensus is needed in the reporting of critical values, and a variety of recommendations have been proposed worldwide (for reviews, see Campbell and Horvath[17,18]). Based on survey studies, tests and critical thresholds are generally chosen from a variety of sources; however, the greatest tendency is toward the use of the published literature and the laboratory's professional experience, often in consultation with clinical staff and manufacturer's recommendations.[17,19,20] Historically, there has been a general lack of outcomes data with respect to critical laboratory values reporting, limiting the ability to choose tests in an evidence-based manner. More recent studies have begun to examine this in more depth, but generalization is difficult because of the heterogeneity of the findings.[9,21,22]

Unlike critical values reported by the clinical pathology laboratory, anatomic pathology findings that require escalated timing of reporting tend to be qualitative rather than quantitative and are relatively rare occurrences (estimated at approximately 0.5% in a retrospective analysis of more than 2700 cases).[23] Because of this, communication of critical values in anatomic pathology is difficult to standardize or even to characterize, and the literature examining this type of communication is exceedingly sparse.

Several survey-based investigations of the concept of critical diagnoses in surgical pathology prompted a closer look at this issue in the literature[7,24] and culminated in the 2006 publication by the Association of Directors of Anatomic and Surgical Pathology (ADASP) of recommendations for critical diagnoses in anatomic pathology.[23] The authors included a table with a list of example critical diagnoses and recommended the development of specific guidelines as an important safety initiative.

More recently, ADASP and the CAP collaboratively published a new set of evidence-based recommendations for dealing with critical diagnoses in anatomic pathology.[6] These recommendations are based on a comprehensive literature search, which identified only nine relevant studies; the overall evidence strength was evaluated as "poor." Recommendations were reviewed further and modified on the basis of public comment on the draft recommendations. Although the final recommendations in this updated publication provide general definitions of *urgent* and *significant and unexpected* diagnoses, they state that each institution should establish and validate its own methods for dealing with the reporting of such diagnoses. Furthermore, the recommendations acknowledge that situations may be unique and difficult to predict, and that determination of urgent and/or significant and unexpected diagnoses depends heavily on clinical judgment.[6]

Unlike the preanalytic and postanalytic phases, errors in the clinical laboratory are much less common in the analytic phase of testing. Although they do occur, errors are limited by rigorous quality control and quality assurance policies developed by laboratories and mandated by various laboratory-accrediting bodies. The error rate of the analytic phase of laboratory medicine has decreased consistently over the past decades and has been recently reported as the lowest in health care at 0.002%.[25]

On the anatomic pathology side, analytic phase error rates are more difficult to pin down. Diagnostic decisions are based mainly on the pathologist's experience and knowledge combined with clinical correlation, and as such they have a subjective component. This is combined with the significant variability of patients' underlying disease processes, potentially causing interpretive differences. Thus, many of the same issues of difficulty with standardization and categorization as discussed above with critical diagnoses apply to this discussion as well. Many studies, discussed throughout this chapter, have investigated error rates in anatomic pathology; however, using error rates to define *quality* is problematic without standardized methods, agreement on types and severity of errors, or, in some cases, agreement on the definition of *error* in the context of the anatomic pathology laboratory.

Some groups have attempted to address these issues. For example, Nakhleh et al[26] focused specifically on the role of case reviews in surgical pathology and cytopathology in an attempt at standardization of, and with an eye toward reducing, interpretive diagnostic errors. The aforementioned evidence-based recommendations from the CAP and ADASP recommended that anatomic pathologists perform timely case reviews relevant to their practice setting, maintain continuous monitoring and documentation, and have procedures in place to improve agreement among diagnosticians.[6] The authors acknowledge that limitations, such as practice settings with only a single pathologist, may limit the implementation of their recommendations.

Despite these challenges, it is clear that errors do occur, and it is worthwhile to work to mitigate them. Typical quality control and quality assurance measures in the anatomic pathology laboratory include some combination of best-practice protocols, intradepartmental and interdepartmental consultations and consensus conferences, cytology-histology and frozen-permanent section correlations, and ongoing education programs.

The above discussion highlights the general importance of information fidelity within laboratories and between clinicians and laboratories. However, transitions of care from one health care provider to another represent a special case of communication in health care and warrant a closer look.

Patient Care Transitions

Over the past decade, communication failures and their effect on patients have been well documented in subspecialties of medicine other than pathology and laboratory medicine, where they have risen to prominence in the literature as one major cause of patient harm. Patient care transitions (called variously in the literature *handoffs*, *sign-offs*, or *hand-overs*) have become more common with the recent advent of resident duty hour restrictions in the United States, particularly in teaching hospital settings; studies investigating their effects have increased concomitantly. The growing realization that communication failures have a dramatic impact on patient safety has prompted regulatory agencies to mandate that institutions adopt ways of organizing information transfer among health care practitioners, which has sweeping implications for all specialties of medicine.

In its *Comprehensive Accreditation Manual for Hospitals*, The Joint Commission includes in its standards a requirement for "a standardized approach to handoff communications."[14] In 2008, The Joint Commission Center for Transforming Healthcare was created to address critical issues of patient safety and propose solutions. Several projects are currently ongoing, one of which is "Handoff Communication"[27] (see also later in that publication, "Tools for Effective Communication"). In 2007, the World Health Organization (although not a regulatory agency per se) teamed with The Joint Commission and Joint Commission International to facilitate worldwide access to tools and strategies to improve patient safety.[28] In addition, specialty-focused and institution-focused guidelines and recommendations have been created (see, for example, the 2012 American College of Obstetricians and Gynecologists Committee opinion,[29] Anderson,[30] and Lane-Fall[31]).

In pathology and laboratory medicine, patient care transitions suffer from a relative paucity of studies explicitly investigating communication issues and their impacts on patient adverse events. These issues can span the total testing process from preanalytic

Communication, Handoffs, and Transitions

through analytic to postanalytic, and when breakdowns occur they carry the potential for patient harm.

Handoff events within clinical pathology tend to occur in situations where direct patient care is likely, such as during the performance of apheresis procedures and the care of patients with possible transfusion reactions. Other situations include direct communications between residents/attending physicians and clinicians concerning specific laboratory testing for patients. No studies have explicitly examined patient care handoffs within this care setting; information must be extrapolated from the literature in other specialties (see later in this chapter).

In anatomic pathology (surgical pathology, cytopathology, and autopsy pathology), the initial information handoff between health care providers is between pathologist and surgeon, interventionalist (endoscopist, radiologist, etc), or clinician. Adequate, pertinent, and accurate clinical information is crucial to the pathologist's ability to provide an accurate and complete diagnosis downstream from this initial communication. For example, clear documentation on accessioning paperwork or in-person communication of special instructions for specimen handling and orientation facilitates the proper processing of surgical specimens so that diagnostic material will be available on the slides for review.

Intraoperatively or during procedures such as fine-needle aspiration, communication between the interventionalist clinician or surgeon and the pathologist can immediately affect patient management. Accurate transfer of the physician's clinical impressions and specific diagnostic questions must be coupled with the pathologist's communication of the diagnosis. Communication errors (as distinct from sampling errors) within these settings have been only sparsely studied. However, in two recent chart review studies, the rate of discordance between pathologists' intraoperative verbal diagnostic rendering and clinicians' reports has been found to be generally low, ranging from 2.7% to 9.6%; and only 0.3% in one study were judged to have more than minimal clinical impact.[32,33]

Particularly in academic settings, resident involvement in pathology cases is significant—residents are intimately involved with and responsible for many steps in the communication chain. Frequently, one resident/attending team is responsible for the frozen section on a specimen, and a different resident will complete the gross description and sign out the case with a different attending. The same may be true in cytopathology, where one resident/attending team assesses specimen adequacy and a second team finalizes the diagnosis. This process becomes even more complex with the rise of personalized medicine and molecular pathology, where even more teams of trainees and attending pathologists become intimately associated with rendering a diagnosis. Steps must be taken to retain the information gleaned directly from the clinician, as well as document the pathologists' (potentially multiple) activities.

The surgical pathology gross description, an evolving skill and an integral part of the resident curriculum, is a mainstay in the effort to maintain continuity of information during the workup of pathology cases. Particularly with complicated specimens, the first-pass effort at the gross description is often supplemented with verbal and interactive communication of findings to the sign-out resident or attending. Continuity is also paramount between outgoing and incoming residents on service or those taking weekend and evening call and needing to assume responsibility for pending cases. This may include specimens with pending special stains or requiring extended fixation or decalcification, and that may require complicated and detailed handoff communications. At our institutions, liberal use is made of diagrams and photographs to prevent loss of information critical to the diagnosis.

A major aspect of the communication of case information occurs between the resident and attending involved in the case. Particularly in later years of training, the resident may have considerable responsibility for specimen handling, and the ability to communicate what was done and why is often critical to the successful rendering of a final diagnosis, which is the end goal of the anatomic pathology service's contribution to good patient care.

Communication is a fluid, back-and-forth process between attending and resident. Ideally, it is embedded in a mentoring relationship with specific goals and expectations for each party, including a system of graduated responsibility for the resident. Good communication necessitates clear and timely feedback from attending to resident, which not only enables effective learning, but also facilitates clear discussions between the resident and other practitioners involved in the patient's care. In pathology and laboratory medicine, the impact of the resident/attending relationship upon patient safety is currently unexamined in the literature; however, studies in other disciplines have shown that breakdowns in communication between attending and resident can lead to patient safety issues.[34,35] Furthermore, perceptions about roles and responsibilities can differ between attending and resident.[36]

At our institutions, residents are often responsible for ensuring that the appropriate clinical information is gleaned from the medical record and communicated to the attending during sign-out. Open lines of communication can facilitate this. Communication of the gross descriptors, as described above, is pertinent to this discussion, along with data obtained from sister services within and outside of the department, such as radiology and flow cytometry.

The last information transfer in the anatomic pathology handoff chain is the communication of the final surgical, cytologic, or autopsy diagnosis. This step may be preceded by a verbal communication of a preliminary diagnosis, particularly when findings qualify as "significant" (see the above discussion of critical diagnoses in anatomic pathology in this chapter). Direct communication with the clinician at this stage can also clarify specific diagnostic questions and expectations for the content of the report, as well as expectations for ancillary testing.

Communication issues relevant to the final surgical pathology report have been well-studied (see Nakhleh[37] for a recent review). In one interesting multidisciplinary example of a study seeking to improve clarity of pathology reports, Valenstein[38] used a literature review from the fields of publishing, aviation, cognitive psychology, and pathology, coupled with a review of 10,000 pathology reports, to derive four general evidence-based principles for report formatting. These include (1) use of diagnostic headlines for emphasis, (2) consistency in layout, (3) decrease in information density for improved readability, and (4) elimination of unnecessary information to remove visual clutter.

Handoff communications are a vital component of patient care, occur systemwide in all medical specialties, and have the broad potential to affect patient safety. Given these facts, it is unsurprising that in recent years the inclusion of formal requirements for patient care transitions in resident education has also become widespread.

Handoffs in Graduate Medical Education

In 2003, the Accreditation Council for Graduate Medical Education (ACGME) defined the maximum hours of work per week for physician trainees, stating: "duty hours must be limited to 80 hours per week, averaged over a four-week period, inclusive of all in-house call activities."[39] In 2011, the ACGME modified this definition to "duty hours must be limited to 80 hours per week, averaged over a four-week period, inclusive of all in-house call activities and all moonlighting."[39] Implicit in the work hour restriction was a need to increase the number of resident shifts and, by extension, patient handoffs between physicians and staff responsible for their care. These changes have raised questions about the effects of increased transitions on patient safety.

As noted earlier in this chapter, The Joint Commission recognized the need to address patient handoffs in the context of the new resident duty hour restrictions and highlighted the need for handoff improvement in their 2006 National Patient Safety Goals. In 2010, The Joint Commission integrated patient handoffs into its accreditation standards, requiring faculty to monitor patient handoffs by trainees.[14] The progressive incorporation of handoffs into The Joint Commission standards highlights the importance of effective handoffs for patient safety.

Several studies have attempted to address how the work hour restrictions affect resident experience and patient safety. One survey of residents and fellows at two large teaching hospitals, which included a subset of pathology trainees, was conducted over 2 years before and after the work hour limits were implemented, to investigate whether perspectives changed with the restrictions. Perception regarding handoffs was included in the assessment, and trainees felt that poor handoff communication contributed to medical errors, both before and after the work hour restrictions were implemented, suggesting that handoffs are a continued perceived area for improvement in patient safety.[40]

Transition of care and teamwork are notably absent in the 2003 ACGME standards but are present in the 2011 update. With regard to transition of care, the new standards require the following five touchstones: (1) that clinical assignments be designed to minimize transitions when possible; (2) that programs monitor transitions to ensure effectiveness; (3) that continuity of care and patient safety be paramount; (4) that trainees be competent in handoffs; and (5) that schedules be available, clearly stating responsible parties at any given time. With regard to teamwork, the standards dictate that patients must be cared for in environments that optimize effective communication, including among the various parts of an interdisciplinary team. There must be a documented process, and examples of how transitions of care can be monitored are offered by the ACGME in a document released in 2011 and updated in 2014, which include reviewing transition-of-care documents and interviewing transitioning team members to ensure that pertinent and correct information is being transferred between the responsible parties.[41]

The Joint Commission and the ACGME offer a guideline for standardization of handoff communication; however, the standards leave much latitude to individual training programs to develop the details of implementation, which leads to diverse approaches that are not necessarily "standard" among institutions. The ACGME also defined specific aspects of the new standards as they apply to different specialties, including pathology. In pathology and laboratory medicine, it is stated that trainees must demonstrate the ability to work with and communicate to health care professionals to provide effective, patient-focused care.[42] However, details are not given as to how this must occur, and there were no distinctions made between anatomic and clinical pathology.

Pathologists comprise multiple subspecialties and form an integral part of the interdisciplinary patient care team. As such, we are critical components of information transfer, requiring effective patient care handoffs at multiple levels. Examples of handoff situations within the pathology discipline include pathology trainee to pathology trainee, pathology trainee to pathology attending, and pathologist to primary clinician. All of these communications and others not explicitly listed must be effective in order to deliver safe patient care.

Handoffs between primary clinicians often include information generated by the laboratory and therefore deserve mention. One example is the handoff between primary clinicians when the patient transitions from inpatient to outpatient status. Any pending test results ordered by the inpatient team need to be appropriately followed by the patient's provider after discharge. Usually this information is relayed in the discharge documentation system because at the time of discharge the follow-up clinician might be unknown.[43] However, if tests are still pending, it could be useful to reference this specific information as well as the party responsible for follow-up, if known. Alerts in the electronic medical record (EMR) are useful; however, the ordering clinician might receive the results, when in fact a different provider has assumed care of the patient by the time the result is available. Alerting the responsible party, and perhaps the patient as well, to the pending results could also be useful to ensure follow-up on those results. An example of how the pathologist can play a vital role is when a patient is discharged home, but a biopsy result is pending. If there is a result that should be acknowledged, the pathologist can step in at this time and ensure the result is received by the appropriate provider, which can help ensure timely care for the patient.

Instances of patient handoff between the pathologist and the primary clinical team are the relay of critical laboratory values, frozen section diagnoses, and diagnostic reports (discussed earlier in this chapter). With regard to pathologist-to-pathologist transfer of information, the trainee working off-hours must be able to effectively communicate information to the pathologist assuming care and vice versa. Because pathology is a diverse specialty, there are many examples of this type of handoff, including patients undergoing evaluation for apheresis, patients undergoing workup for transfusion-related issues or acute leukemia, and specimens processed after hours that need further attention by the primary pathology service.

Approximately 20% to 30% of information in handoffs does not appear in the documented medical record. Patient handoffs are highly variable, and potential consequences of inadequate patient handoffs include but are not limited to adverse events, delays in diagnosis and treatment, redundant events (such as tests), longer hospital stays, higher cost, and less effective medical education. The role of the laboratory can affect several of these factors, and one of the main purposes of specimen triage in clinical laboratories is to try to prevent these consequences.[44]

Few studies directly address handoffs within pathology and laboratory medicine or between pathology and other medical specialties. The Joint Commission standards are applicable to all specialties, and therefore the information gleaned thus far in studies regarding patient handoffs must be extrapolated until there is a richer peer-reviewed and validated literature in the field of pathology. Strategies applied to patient handoffs in other specialties might be adaptable to fit the needs of our discipline, and some of these are alluded to below, with an emphasis on application to the field.

Incorporating Handoffs Into Medical Education

The ACGME recommendations that went into effect in 2011 included a requirement that faculty monitor resident handoffs[40]; however, there are no clear guidelines on how to implement this responsibility, and there is room for interpretation in curriculum development. Strategies that are already being implemented in other specialties (eg, pediatrics), as well as at different levels of training, are potentially applicable to pathology and laboratory medicine resident education.

In 2010, the Association for Computing Machinery hosted a symposium entitled, "Handovers and Handoffs: Collaborating in Turns," with a goal of developing tools and resources for effective medical education regarding patient handoffs. Wohlauer and colleagues[45] attempted to clarify the definition of patient handoffs, emphasizing the transfer of information and responsibility between both participants, which must involve a shared understanding. Issues in patient handoffs can signify a breakdown in communication, and formal training in patient handoffs could, they argued, help prevent this by providing tools and resources to providers.

They propose a blueprint allowing trainees to progress through the ACGME milestones and display competency in all six areas designated by the

Table 4-1. An Approach to the Standardization and Measurement of Patient Handoffs		
Proposed Frame	**Goal**	**Proposed Quality Measure**
(1) Information processing	More effective transfer of data with a standard handoff protocol	Assessment of accuracy of essential content transferred
(2) Stereotypical narratives	Predictable handoff structures that emphasize deviations from *normal*	Assessment of presence of necessary components in the handoff
(3) Resilience	Transparency of one's thought process so that errors or incorrect assumptions can be caught and corrected in real time	Assessment of collaborative cross-checking
(4) Accountability	Alignment of assignment and responsibility focused on transfer of authority to make decisions	Completion of tasks and appropriateness of transferred tasks
(5) Social interactions	Team-based nature of handoffs	Assessment of perceived quality of interpersonal communications
(6) Distributed cognition	Continuous coordinated care that encompasses understanding of a patient's entire clinical situation, across disciplines	Assessment of effectiveness of coordination of care
(7) Cultural norms	"Climate change" interventions for trainees and other individuals who perform patient handoffs	Implementation of policies, procedures, and education

Adapted from Patterson and Wears.[44]

ACGME: patient care, medical knowledge, interpersonal and communication skills, professionalism, practice-based learning and improvement, and systems-based practice.[45] Because residents are now evaluated by this system as they advance through their training programs, assessing handoffs in a universal and familiar way, and making this a standard strategy to do so, could prove useful across time and specialty.

Patterson and Wears[44] took a different approach to address patient handoffs, in the form of seven primary functions (referred to as *framing*). They proposed that the frames could be used to develop tools and quality measures, including policies, procedures, and educational objectives inserted into the curriculum at multiple levels in the health care system. The seven proposed primary frames, with the goal and proposed quality measure for each, are outlined in Table 4-1.

Regardless of the approach, it is clear that, at the very least, there must be a way to hand off patient information and care in a consistent manner. Strategies proposed for formal training in handoffs might include several approaches, including a sequestered time during orientation, integration into EMRs, and, perhaps most popularly, mnemonics. There are also temporal considerations to consider. Residents need to be competent in handoffs from the day they start training, and some authors argue that handoff education should begin in medical school. A survey of third-year medical students at two US schools reported that medical students often participate in handoffs at some level, and the authors emphasized the importance of this in the medical students' increasing confidence to hand off patient information as they mature in the system.[46]

A handoff curriculum was instituted at the Medical University of South Carolina and included a formalized handoff training day during orientation for incoming postgraduate year (PGY) -1 trainees. This day involved a didactic session (using tools such as mnemonics), small group sessions, and simulated handoffs. A potential advantage of this is to introduce a universal approach for handoffs and to allow for intervention and constructive criticism before the involvement of real patients.[47]

Other approaches involve implementation and development of everyday tools for trainees, such as a variety of mnemonic memory aids. One example is the PACT (Priority, Admissions, Changes, and Tasks) mnemonic, as well as others discussed elsewhere.[48] Other tools include standardized handoff systems including checklist formats, electronic templates, and other tools based on the EMR.[30,49-51] A study assessing the impact of an electronic template in the patient handoff concluded that use of a template was associated with an increase in handoff content—specifically the active problem list, clinical status, and anticipatory guidance—and a decrease in data omissions. There was a trend toward reduction in near-miss events; however, the data did not reach statistical significance.[50]

The Veterans Affairs system designed and implemented a physician-to-physician handoff tool based on the EMR, which has now been incorporated into the entire Veterans Affairs system.[30] Another approach to education is to implement simulations. One preintervention and postintervention pilot study used a simulated operating room in which handoffs could be performed after a 1-day course in simulation-based handoffs. The simulated handoffs were again observed 1 year after initial training, and decreases in omissions and errors were observed.[52]

Although some of the studies suggested that incorporation of tools into handoffs could be useful, an important point to address is whether the tools are actually effective. Starmer et al[53] conducted a prospective study in multiple pediatric residency programs to assess the impact of a handoff program, which included a mnemonic, training, faculty development and observation program, and a sustainability campaign. The mnemonic, I-PASS (Illness severity, Patient summary, Action items, Situation awareness and contingency plans, and Synthesis by receiver), is trademarked by Boston Children's Hospital (materials freely available) and was incorporated into the EMR in several of the institutions involved in the study. Implementation of the handoff program resulted in a decrease in the medical error rate by 23% and a decrease in the preventable adverse events by 30%.[53] Other programs and specialties are now looking into adoption of the approach.[31]

Despite the potential of handoff tools to increase effectiveness of patient handoffs, concerns remain. First, any and all handoff systems are inherently dependent on the presumption that the information transferred is up-to-date and accurate, and this responsibility ultimately rests on the individuals performing the handoff.[51] Second, in order to improve handoffs, the system in which the handoffs occur must be organized so that providers are properly armed with the education and the tools needed to implement handoffs accurately and effectively.[54] Third, there is a growing concern that despite the many new tools, handoffs could become "too automatic," potentially leading to new, unanticipated errors.[55] One instance of this is the ability of physicians to copy and paste patient notes in electronic systems. Patient care evolves over time; however, this is not always apparent when reading EMRs, which have been copied with minimal changes. Even if updates are present in the note, repetition of older and potentially no longer relevant text can lead to the potential for overlooking important changes and updates. Suggestions to avoid falling into this potential trap include the use of handoff systems such as SBAR (discussed later in this chapter), which provides a general structure within which open communication is allowed for engaged discussions regarding patient care and complete understanding of the information being transferred.[55]

In addition, Nuckols and Escarce[56] attest that cost must be considered when implementing different handoff strategies. One potential cost is having a computerized handoff system, which is estimated to be up to $60,000 at large institutions. A second consideration is potential increase in resident labor and time when using structured sign-outs, especially for programs that do not already have a structured sign-out in place and must build or purchase and then implement one.[56] Investment in the development of handoff systems could actually be a cost-saving strategy in the long run because implicit in the goals of improvement of patient care and patient outcomes is less cost to the patient and to the health care system overall. Despite the concern of automaticity, cost, and unanticipated adverse effects, handoffs are now considered an essential part of health care, and proper execution of handoffs should be considered the norm in health care and therefore health care education.

Handoffs in Pathology Graduate Medical Education

In the discipline of pathology, several layers of patient handoffs must be considered involving physicians, laboratory technologists, who play a vital role in sample processing and results generation, and nurses involved in procedures. Residents on different pathology services transfer information throughout the day. Residents often communicate any potential issues to the covering resident taking call overnight, and, conversely, the covering resident taking call overnight transfers pending issues to the relevant service the next day. Any communication that occurs off hours will inherently occur between the covering residents on both ends of the discussion.

The backbone of pathology and laboratory medicine involves the laboratories providing test results and interpretations to clinicians (including other pathologists), and laboratories are often continuously operational. The observation that approximately 60% to 70% of medical decisions are based on laboratory results clearly emphasizes the importance of the laboratory in patient care. Hence, effective handoffs at shift change between laboratory personnel are also an essential component of continuity of care. Laboratories are complex systems and highly regulated, but little information is known regarding handoffs in this setting. An institution in the Netherlands developed a system that involves a standard checklist used at each shift change. The components of the checklist are as follows: (1) current state of laboratory staffing, (2) information technology issues, (3) technical issues,

(4) analytical issues, (5) nonconformities, (6) service level, (7) patient cases for handoff, and (8) interesting cases for continuing education.[57] Development of such standard handoffs in clinical laboratories could prove useful, and further research could be beneficial.

Information must also be passed between subspecialties in pathology in an effective manner both during daytime hours and during overnight call. Certain pathology subspecialties, such as hematopathology, require real-time transfer of information as well as specimens for ancillary testing. The Hospital of the University of Pennsylvania has developed a custom database with dashboards, which facilitates transfer of information, allowing for more effective communication and documentation of hematopathology specimen triage.[58] Residents taking overnight call could utilize a system of verbal and/or written communication to transfer information to the relevant service for follow-up during daytime hours.

Communication of diagnoses between pathology services and primary clinicians occurs primarily through written reports, and clear and concise writing can facilitate effective information transfer. Particularly as genetic testing becomes more prevalent, integration of molecular genetic testing results in a comprehensive report can simplify effective communication of results to the clinician. Scheuner et al[59] created a molecular pathology report template combining synoptic and narrative formats, with information grouped to flow in a logical manner. The reports were structured to include the following components: (1) patient information, (2) physician information, (3) test performed, (4) test results, (5) test interpretation, (6) guidance on next steps (if applicable), and (7) supplemental information. The overall intention was to streamline and standardize the reporting process, so that relevant information could be communicated and further discussion could be encouraged when warranted. They implemented molecular pathology templates into their reporting system and subsequently surveyed clinicians about their perception of the communication of results. Development of a standardized template utilizing a combined synoptic and narrative format was well received and improved clinician satisfaction.[60]

Communication gaps are a component of missed laboratory results and misinformation.[61] Smith et al[62] encouraged the clinical team to assign specific staff to follow up on such results and also encouraged the clinical laboratory to be active in its role to convey results when possible. The communication must be of sound quality to ensure the most effective patient care possible, and there are some essential components to ensure effective communication.

Key Requirements for Effective Communication

For handoffs to be effective and successful, they should possess certain qualities. The American College of Obstetricians and Gynecologists published a committee opinion in 2012 stating that effective handoffs should have interactive communications, limited interruptions, a process for verification, and an opportunity to review any relevant historical data.[29] Interactive communications imply a bidirectional exchange; however, the exchange should be beneficial to both parties, and taking certain factors into account could have an impact on quality. Language must be considered, especially with verbal handoffs. Awareness of potential language barriers, including medical jargon, can be helpful to avoid scenarios where miscommunication occurs due to misunderstanding of the words used to communicate. Clarifying questions and phonetic spelling could help eliminate these language barriers. Although many handoffs are electronic, this is not universal, and handwritten communication is still a common practice. Illegible handwriting, particularly in acute clinical situations, can also lead to miscommunication. Encouragement of print or otherwise legible handwriting could be useful. One suggestion to limit interruptions is to provide an isolated environment free of distractions and that permits confidentiality. Clarifying and acknowledging transfer of responsibility between care providers is also critical when transfer of information occurs. Standardization of communication methods can help establish a routine, which can facilitate communication transfer between health care providers.

The field of aviation utilizes "readbacks" extensively between pilots and air traffic controllers, and is very successful (though not infallible); this method has been applied to the health care setting in general as well as to pathology.[63] Implementation of readbacks has been incorporated into health care in an effort to render patient handoffs and verbal communication more effective. The Joint Commission requires that staff use a record and readback process before taking action on a verbal order or verbal report of a critical result. Providers in pathology and laboratory medicine must ensure that the record and readback occurs and is documented properly.[64] The readback system involves a back-and-forth communication between involved parties. Information is given from the first party to the second, who processes the information and reads it back. The first party then processes the readback, and the communication loop is closed and documented. Actions are then taken on the basis of this communication.

Implementation of readbacks, phonetic spelling, and clarifying questions can all contribute to an improvement in transfer of patient information. The system of readbacks is still subject to errors, and several scenarios can be imagined in which errors might occur. Correct information might be given but not received, and therefore read back incorrectly. Correct information might be given and read back (and therefore presumed received and understood), but actions taken after the readback might be incorrect. Correct information might be given, received, and read back, but the documentation and loop closure might not occur correctly. When applied to pathology, readbacks have been proposed to have an important role in communication of critical values, frozen section diagnoses, and patient handoffs. In some institutions, critical values can be called to clinical pathology residents when other physicians cannot be reached in a timely manner. This adds an additional person to the communication loop. Frozen section diagnoses are often called to operating rooms, typically using a speaker system; however, sometimes nurses, surgical assistants, or other health care personnel are "answering the phone," and their understanding of the subtleties of the diagnosis may be misunderstood or misinterpreted; for example, failing to recognize the *in situ* portion of the phrase *carcinoma in situ*. Accurate data communication in these settings is critical because it can change real-time patient management, and there are tools that can help facilitate handoffs.

Tools for Effective Communication

In order to address and improve quality in handoffs, tools are available to help with the system as well as with the details. The Joint Commission has established with nine participating institutions a project called, Joint Commission Center for Transforming Healthcare.[65] This group is developing a handoff communications Targeted Solutions Tool (TST), with the goal of making handoff tools widely available to the more than 20,000 health care organizations accredited by The Joint Commission. The strategy is to identify potential problems with handoffs and develop solutions to specifically target problem areas. Handoffs are described as the transfer of information involving a sender of information and a receiver of information. Problems identified are divided into three categories: (1) general—culture, expectations, timing, interruptions, lack of standardized procedure, staffing, and so forth; (2) sending—sender provides inaccurate or incomplete information, unable to contact receiver of information, and so forth; and (3) receiving—unaware of handoff, inability to follow up, lack of knowledge of information gaps, and so forth.

A few examples can illustrate how the TST tool might work in practice. Within the *general* category, an institution may recognize a need for systemic cultural change in order to improve handoff effectiveness. The targeted solutions for this cultural change may include ensuring that handoffs are an educational priority and performance expectation, standardizing handoffs at the institutional level, and engaging staff to improve their handoffs by giving real-time feedback. Examples of targeting communication methods for the *sender* and *receiver* to improve communication include implementation of handoff tools, some of which are discussed elsewhere in this chapter.

The acronym SHARE has been developed by the Joint Commission Center for Transforming Healthcare to address issues and targeted solutions. Above are some examples, but this proposed process is designed to be used universally to allow for continued improvement in patient handoffs.[65]

> The *S* is for Standardization of critical content. The sender of information should provide the receiver with relevant patient information, and synthesize and emphasize pertinent and critical elements of the information from all sources, so that the receiver gets a concise and succinct summary of the patient and can comfortably assume responsibility for the patient.
>
> The *H* is for Hardwire within your system. This addresses the need for the institution to develop and implement a standardized handoff method for universal use within the system, establishing a physical environment conducive to sending and receiving patient handoffs, having protected time, and clearly stating expectations for patient handoffs, with the goal of ideally instituting cultural changes that promote safe and effective handoffs.
>
> The *A* is for Allowing opportunity to ask questions. This is not always easy when considering time constraints, but allowing some time to digest patient information and clarify why something is happening if it is not clear is critical to safe patient care.
>
> The *R* is for Reinforcement of quality and measurement. Development and utilization of a system to measure handoffs is essential for identifying problem areas in an institution and monitoring patient handoffs (as is now required as part of training and The Joint Commission standards), and it is also a way to track improvements.

Allowing the people who are actively using the handoff system to see the results and impact of their efforts is a great motivator.

The *E* is for Educate and coach. Education of staff at the start of training, as well as whenever changes are made to the system, is key. Ensuring that staff are aware of expectations and requirements is essential to implementation of a successful handoff system. Continuing education, such as giving feedback in real time, can allow health care personnel to revisit fundamental concepts, make improvements, and identify areas where the system can be improved.[65]

The American Medical Association has a webpage dedicated to resources for improving patient handoffs, including several mnemonics, which could prove useful in a variety of settings, including pathology and laboratory medicine. One popular system is the SBAR system, which was originally developed by the US Navy, which has been applied to the health care setting and expanded into the ISBARQ acronym.[66, 67]

The *I* is for Identify (ie, the specific person or people caring for the patient), and the goal is to clarify the roles and responsibilities of those involved in a patient care handoff.

The *S* is for Situation and indicates the need for the personnel assuming care to acclimate to the patient's current state.

The *B* is for Background, and the aim is to provide relevant and up-to-date medical information on the patient.

The *A* is for Assessment, and this includes the impression of the patient and of the situation by the provider handing off the information, as well as anticipated needs.

The *R* is for Recommendation and signifies the need for transmission of adequate knowledge of the patient's treatment plan going forward. This includes pending laboratory results, pending studies, and the patient's anticipated status at the next handoff.

The *Q* is for Questions and answers, and this is to promote bidirectional communication between the parties conducting the handoff.[67]

The ISBARQ system is likely to be used in some form in many handoff situations, but applying a standard system might help promote consistency, especially because handoffs often occur in error-prone situations. In particular, the ISBARQ system could be applied to many situations in pathology and laboratory medicine, including but not limited to change of shift to and from the pathology residents on call.

Verbal handoffs have been likened to the game of telephone, where the message degrades with each subsequent communication, potentially resulting in a message that is different from the original. Applying this analogy to the communication of patient care highlights the vulnerability of the system to errors and the potential of the many available communication tools to improve patient safety.[67]

As pathologists, we are not just an ancillary service providing results to clinicians. We are physicians who use our medical training to interpret findings, and we strive to communicate them in a meaningful way. Development of tools within pathology and laboratory medicine designed to address the unique issues we encounter in our specialty and various subspecialties could prove invaluable to improvement of communication with colleagues across all disciplines in addition to our own.

References

1. Kohn LT, Corrigan JM, Donaldson MS, eds; Committee on Quality of Health Care in America; Institute of Medicine. *To Err is Human: Building a Safer Health System*. Washington, DC: National Academy Press; 2000.
2. Richardson WC, Berwick DM, Bisgard JC, eds; Committee on Quality of Health Care in America; Institute of Medicine. *Crossing the Quality Chasm: A New Health System for the 21st Century*. Washington, DC: National Academy Press; 2001.
3. Institute of Medicine Committee on Quality of Health Care in America. *Improving Diagnosis in Health Care*. Washington, DC: National Academies Press; 2015.
4. Wagar EA, Horowitz RE, Siegal GP. *Laboratory Administration for Pathologists*. Northfield, IL: College of American Pathologists; 2011.
5. Tworek JA, Volmar KE, McCall SJ, et al. Q-Probes studies in anatomic pathology: quality improvement through targeted benchmarking. *Arch Pathol Lab Med*. 2014;138(9):1156-1166.
6. Nakhleh RE, Myers JL, Allen TC, et al. Consensus statement on effective communication of urgent diagnoses and significant, unexpected diagnoses in surgical pathology and cytopathology from the College of American Pathologists and Association of Directors of Anatomic and Surgical Pathology. *Arch Pathol Lab Med*. 2012;136(2):148-154.
7. Pereira TC, Silverman JF, LiVolsi V, et al. A multi-institutional survey of critical diagnoses (critical values) in surgical pathology and cytology. *Am J Clin Pathol*. 2008;130(5):731-735.
8. Smith LB. Pathology review of outside material: when does it help and when can it hurt? *J Clin Oncol*. 2011;29(19):2724-2727.
9. Piva E, Pelloso M, Penello L, et al. Laboratory critical values: automated notification supports effective clinical decision making. *Clin Biochem*. 2014;47(13-14):1163-1168.

10. Grimm E, Friedberg RC, Wilkinson DS, et al. Blood bank safety practices: mislabeled samples and wrong blood in tube: a Q-Probes analysis of 122 clinical laboratories. *Arch Pathol Lab Med*. 2010;134(8):1108-1115.
11. Nakhleh RE, Idowu MO, Souers RJ, et al. Mislabeling of cases, specimens, blocks, and slides: a College of American Pathologists study of 136 institutions. *Arch Pathol Lab Med*. 2011;135(8):969-974.
12. Hammond ME, Hayes DF, Dowsett M, et al. American Society of Clinical Oncology/College of American Pathologists guideline recommendations for immunohistochemical testing of estrogen and progesterone receptors in breast cancer. *Arch Pathol Lab Med*. 2010;134(6):907-922.
13. Lundberg GD. When to panic over an abnormal value. *MLO Med Lab Obs*. 1972;4:47-54.
14. National Patient Safety Goals Effective January 1, 2015. The Joint Commission. http://www.jointcommission.org/assets/1/6/2015_NPSG_HAP.pdf. Accessed April 28, 2016.
15. Clinical Laboratory Improvement Amendments of 1988. Part 493. Laboratory Requirements. http://www.ecfr.gov/cgi-bin/text-idx?SID=1248e3189da5e5f936e-55315402bc38b&node=pt42.5.493&rgn=div5. Accessed April 28, 2016.
16. Singh H, Vij MS. Eight recommendations for policies for communicating abnormal test results. *Jt Comm J Qual Patient Saf*. 2010;36(5):226-232.
17. Campbell C, Horvath A. Towards harmonisation of critical laboratory result management: review of the literature and survey of Australasian practices. *Clin Biochem Rev*. 2012;33(4):149-160.
18. Campbell CA, Horvath AR. Harmonization of critical result management in laboratory medicine. *Clin Chim Acta*. 2014;432:135-147.
19. Howanitz PJ, Steindel SJ, Heard NV. Laboratory critical values policies and procedures: a College of American Pathologists Q-Probes Study in 623 institutions. *Arch Pathol Lab Med*. 2002;126(6):663-669.
20. Wagar EA, Friedberg RC, Souers R, et al. Critical values comparison: a College of American Pathologists Q-Probes survey of 163 clinical laboratories. *Arch Pathol Lab Med*. 2007;131(12):1769-1775.
21. Doering TA, Plapp F, Crawford JM. Establishing an evidence base for critical laboratory value thresholds. *Am J Clin Pathol*. 2014;142(5):617-628.
22. Jenkins JJ, Mac Crawford J, Bissell MG. Studying critical values: adverse event identification following a critical laboratory values study at the Ohio State University Medical Center. *Am J Clin Pathol*. 2007;128(4):604-609.
23. Silverman JF, Pereira TC. Critical values in anatomic pathology. *Arch Pathol Lab Med*. 2006;130(5):638-640.
24. Nakhleh RE, Souers R, Brown RW. Significant and unexpected, and critical diagnoses in surgical pathology: a College of American Pathologists' survey of 1130 laboratories. *Arch Pathol Lab Med*. 2009;133(9):1375-1378.
25. Hawkins R. Managing the pre- and post-analytical phases of the total testing process. *Ann Lab Med*. 2012;32(1):5-16.
26. Nakhleh RE, Nosé V, Colasacco C, et al. Interpretive diagnostic error reduction in surgical pathology and cytology: guideline from the College of American Pathologists Pathology and Laboratory Quality Center and the Association of Directors of Anatomic and Surgical Pathology. *Arch Pathol Lab Med*. 2016;140(1):29-40.
27. Project detail: Hand-off communications. The Joint Commission Center for Transforming Healthcare. http://www.centerfortransforminghealthcare.org/projects/detail.aspx?Project=1. Accessed April 28, 2016.
28. Patient safety: WHO Collaborating Centre on Patient Safety Solutions. World Health Organization. http://www.who.int/patientsafety/solutions/patientsafety/collaborating_centre/en/. Accessed April 28, 2016.
29. ACOG Committee Opinion No. 517: Communication strategies for patient handoffs. *Obstet Gynecol*. 2012;119(2 Pt 1):408-411.
30. Anderson J, Shroff D, Curtis A, et al. The Veterans Affairs shift change physician-to-physician handoff project. *Jt Comm J Qual Patient Saf*. 2010;36(2):62-71.
31. Lane-Fall MB, Brooks AK, Wilkins SA, et al. Addressing the mandate for hand-off education: a focused review and recommendations for anesthesia resident curriculum development and evaluation. *Anesthesiology*. 2014;120(1):218-229.
32. Roy S, Parwani AV, Dhir R, et al. Frozen section diagnosis: is there discordance between what pathologists say and what surgeons hear? *Am J Clin Pathol*. 2013;140(3):363-369.
33. Talmon G, Horn A, Wedel W, et al. How well do we communicate?: a comparison of intraoperative diagnoses listed in pathology reports and operative notes. *Am J Clin Pathol*. 2013;140(5):651-657.
34. Kilminster S, Cottrell D, Grant J, et al. AMEE Guide No. 27: Effective educational and clinical supervision. *Med Teach*. 2007;29(1):2-19.
35. Ulmer C, Wolman DM, Johns MME, eds. *Resident Duty Hours: Enhancing Sleep, Supervision, and Safety*. Washington, DC: The National Academies Press; 2008. http://www.nap.edu/catalog/12508/resident-duty-hours-enhancing-sleep-supervision-and-safety. Accessed April 28, 2016.
36. Loo L, Puri N, Kim DI, et al. "Page me if you need me": the hidden curriculum of attending-resident communication. *J Grad Med Educ*. 2012;4(3):340-345.
37. Nakhleh RE. Quality in surgical pathology communication and reporting. *Arch Pathol Lab Med*. 2011;135(11):1394-1397.
38. Valenstein PN. Formatting pathology reports: applying four design principles to improve communication and patient safety. *Arch Pathol Lab Med*. 2008;132(1):84-94.
39. Resident duty hours in the learning and working environment: comparison of 2003 and 2011 standards. Accreditation Council for Graduate Medical Education. https://www.acgme.org/acgmeweb/Portals/0/PDFs/dh-ComparisonTable2003v2011.pdf. Accessed April 28, 2016.

40. Jagsi R, Weinstein DF, Shapiro J, Kitch BT, Dorer D, Weissman JS. The Accreditation Council for Graduate Medical Education's limits on residents' work hours and patient safety. *Arch Intern Med*. 2008;168(5):493-500.
41. Frequently asked questions: ACGME common duty hour requirements. Effective July 1, 2011. Accreditation Council for Graduate Medical Education. https://www.acgme.org/acgmeweb/Portals/0/PDFs/dh-faqs2011.pdf. Updated June 18, 2014. Accessed April 28, 2016.
42. Specialty-specific duty hour definitions. Accreditation Council for Graduate Medical Education. http://www.acgme.org/acgmeweb/portals/0/pdfs/dh_definitions.pdf. Updated October 2015. Accessed April 28, 2016.
43. JCAHO's 2006 National Patient Safety Goals: handoffs are biggest challenge. *Hosp Peer Rev*. 2005;30(7):89-93.
44. Patterson ES, Wears RL. Patient handoffs: standardized and reliable measurement tools remain elusive. *Jt Comm J Qual Patient Saf*. 2010;36(2):52-61.
45. Wohlauer MV, Arora VM, Horwitz LI, et al. The patient handoff: a comprehensive curricular blueprint for resident education to improve continuity of care. *Acad Med*. 2012;87(4):411-418.
46. Arora VM, Eastment MC, Bethea ED, Farnan JM, Friedman ES. Participation and experience of third-year medical students in handoffs: time to sign out? *J Gen Intern Med*. 2013;28(8):994-998.
47. Allen S, Caton C, Cluver J, Mainous AG III, Clyburn B. Targeting improvements in patient safety at a large academic center: an institutional handoff curriculum for graduate medical education. *Acad Med*. 2014;89(10):1366-1369.
48. Tapia NM, Fallon SC, Brandt ML, Scott BG, Suliburk JW. Assessment and standardization of resident handoff practices: PACT project. *J Surg Res*. 2013;184(1):71-77.
49. Abraham J, Kannampallil T, Patel B, Almoosa K, Patel VL. Ensuring patient safety in care transitions: an empirical evaluation of a handoff intervention tool. *AMIA Annu Symp Proc*. 2012;2012:17-26.
50. Graham KL, Marcantonio ER, Huang GC, Yang J, Davis RB, Smith CC. Effect of a systems intervention on the quality and safety of patient handoffs in an internal medicine residency program. *J Gen Intern Med*. 2013;28(8):986-993.
51. Wayne JD, Tyagi R, Reinhardt G, et al. Simple standardized patient handoff system that increases accuracy and completeness. *J Surg Educ*. 2008;65(6):476-485.
52. Pukenas EW, Dodson G, Deal ER, Gratz I, Allen E, Burden AR. Simulation-based education with deliberate practice may improve intraoperative handoff skills: a pilot study. *J Clin Anesth*. 2014;26(7):530-538.
53. Starmer AJ, Spector ND, Srivastava R, et al. Changes in medical errors after implementation of a handoff program. *N Engl J Med*. 2014;371:1803-1812.
54. Van Eaton E. Handoff improvement: we need to understand what we are trying to fix. *Jt Comm J Qual Patient Saf*. 2010;36(2):51.
55. Are handoffs too 'automatic'? QI experts fear errors could rise. *Healthcare Benchmarks Qual Improv*. 2006;13(1):1-4.
56. Nuckols T, Escarce JJ. ACGME Common Program Requirements: potential cost implications of changes to resident duty hours and related changes to the training environment announced on September 28, 2010. Accreditation Council for Graduate Medical Education. https://www.acgme.org/acgmeweb/Portals/0/PDFs/dh-FinalReportCostAnalysis2011CPRs.pdf. Accessed April 28, 2016.
57. de Jonge N, Ballieux BE, Schenk PW, Cobbaert CM. Structured handoff at shift change in a clinical laboratory increases patient safety. *Clin Chem Lab Med*. 2013;51(6):e127-e128.
58. Azzato EM, Morrissette JJD, Halbiger RD, Bagg A, Daber RD. Development and implementation of a custom integrated database with dashboards to assist with hematopathology specimen triage and traffic. *J Pathol Inform*. 2014;5:29.
59. Scheuner MT, Hilborne L, Brown J, Lubin IM; members of the RAND Molecular Genetic Test Report Advisory Board. A report template for molecular genetic tests designed to improve communication between the clinician and laboratory. *Genet Test Mol Biomarkers*. 2012;16(7):761-769.
60. Scheuner MT, Edelen MO, Hilborne LH, Lubin IM; RAND Molecular Genetic Test Report Advisory Board. Effective communication of molecular genetic test results to primary care providers. *Genet Med*. 2013;15(6):444-449.
61. JCAHO's 2006 National Patient Safety Goals: handoffs are biggest challenge. *Hosp Peer Rev*. 2005;30(7):89-93.
62. Smith ML, Raab SS, Fernald DH, et al. Evaluating the connections between primary care practice and clinical laboratory testing: a review of the literature and call for laboratory involvement in the solutions. *Arch Pathol Lab Med*. 2013;137(1):120-125.
63. Prabhakar H, Cooper JB, Sabel A, Weckbach S, Mehler PS, Stahel PF. Introducing standardized "readbacks" to improve patient safety in surgery: a prospective survey in 92 providers at a public safety-net hospital. *BMC Surg*. 2012;12:8.
64. "What did the doctor say?": improving health literacy to protect patient safety. The Joint Commission. http://www.jointcommission.org/assets/1/18/improving_health_literacy.pdf. 2007. Accessed April 28, 2016.
65. Improving transitions of care: hand-off communications. Joint Commission Center for Transforming Healthcare. http://www.centerfortransforminghealthcare.org/assets/4/6/handoff_comm_storyboard.pdf. Updated December 22, 2014. Accessed April 28, 2016.
66. Patient handoffs: resources on improving patient handoffs. The American Medical Association. http://www.ama-assn.org/ama/pub/about-ama/our-people/member-groups-sections/resident-fellow-section/rfs-resources/patient-handoffs.page. Accessed April 28, 2016.
67. Eberhardt S. Improve handoff communication with SBAR. *Nursing*. 2014;44(11):17-20.

5

Utilizing Technology to Improve Laboratory Patient Safety

Anand S. Dighe, MD, PhD

Introduction

Progress over the past two decades has resulted in technology to improve patient safety that is available for use throughout the laboratory testing cycle. The preanalytic phase of testing accounts for 30% to 70% of laboratory errors, many of which have patient safety impacts.[1-3] Common root causes for many of these preanalytic errors are the use of manual, highly variable processes, including paper requisitions, manual registration, sample collection, and manual data entry. Properly deployed, technology can be an important tool to help prevent preanalytic error. In the preanalytic phase, computerized provider order entry, decision support, laboratory information systems, barcoding, and bedside positive patient identification systems can all contribute to improved patient safety.

In the analytic phase, the current generation of laboratory instruments have a variety of built-in error-checking features. In addition, advances in laboratory automation, autoverification, expert systems, interpretive comments, instrument interfacing, dashboards, rules, and middleware can be utilized to minimize error and patient safety risk. In the postanalytic phase, there are numerous opportunities for patient safety errors due to the failure to effectively communicate results, failure to review results, and the misinterpretation of results. The laboratory can use technology to reduce these risks with a variety of techniques including interpretive comments, result monitoring, critical result reporting, and auditing procedures.

In this chapter, an overview of the role of technology to improve patient safety in these three key phases of laboratory testing will be provided. In addition, there are sections covering the patient safety aspects of several areas with unique patient safety concerns that may be addressable by technology, including point-of-care testing, blood transfusion, and anatomic pathology.

Preanalytic Phase

Test Selection

The selection of tests is an error-prone step in the overall testing process.[4-6] Errors in test selection include ordering the wrong tests and failing to order the appropriate tests (Table 5-1). Patients are put at risk by incorrect test selection because inappropriate test orders may lead to overdiagnosis or delayed diagnosis. In the past two decades, the emergence of genomic assays and an array of new diagnostic technologies have been driving an increase in the size and complexity of the laboratory test menu. Moreover, the challenge of test selection is compounded by increasingly busy clinicians with decreased time for each appointment and patient.[7]

Computerized Provider Order Entry

Computerized provider order entry (CPOE) systems permit providers to electronically input orders for laboratory tests, medications, radiology, and other studies. In the United States, the use of CPOE in all care settings is becoming ubiquitous, in part as a result of federal "meaningful use" legislation that

Table 5-1. Technology for Patient Safety in the Preanalytic Phase

Patient Safety Issue	Technology Solution(s)
Manual order transcription	• CPOE with order communication
Missed or incorrect tests	• CPOE ordering templates • CPOE corollary orders • Decision support–based alerts • Enhanced CPOE search functionality
Patient identification errors	• CPOE with order communication • Barcoded patient wristbands
Specimen mislabeling	• CPOE with order communication • Barcoded specimen labels created at bedside using specimen collection systems with positive patient identification • Automated preanalytic processing and aliquotting
Specimen collection problems	• CPOE order comments viewable on bedside collection devices
Timed specimens	• Decision support to link collection of timed specimens to medication administration

CPOE, computerized provider order entry.

provides financial incentives for the adoption and use of CPOE systems.[8] Before the widespread use of CPOE, clinical laboratories generally maintained control over the design of paper requisitions.[9] Paper requisition–based testing panels and predefined order sets offered key tools to guide test selection because many of these panels and order sets essentially encoded laboratory expertise into the work process. With the implementation of CPOE, the laboratory is at risk of losing control over the display of tests and panels because at many institutions the overall CPOE system may be maintained by a central information technology group or by clinical departments other than pathology. To retain influence on this critical part of the test-ordering process, the laboratory must be actively involved in the implementation and maintenance of laboratory CPOE.[10,11]

Even before consideration of the benefits in providing a platform for clinical decision support (CDS), the core features of most CPOE systems have the potential to improve the overall quality and safety of the total testing process by improving order accuracy, eliminating manual processes, and reducing test turnaround time.[12-14] When the correct tests are performed in a rapid manner, there is benefit to a wide variety of workflow and patient outcomes due to eliminating bottlenecks in care and delays in diagnosis. CPOE systems, particularly those with direct electronic transmission of test orders to the laboratory information system (LIS), eliminate error-prone paper requisitions and numerous other manual steps. Paper requisitions, in addition to requiring increased processing time, are particularly susceptible to error and misinterpretation. Tests requested on paper may be missed by the laboratory, or ambiguous/illegible handwritten orders may lead to errors. For example, an electronic CPOE order that is directly transmitted to the LIS with the LIS code for "anti-tissue transglutaminase IgA" (a test for celiac disease) is unambiguous, whereas a paper-based write-in order for "celiac serology" is subject to misinterpretation and delay. It is important to note that CPOE does not necessarily eliminate write-in orders, because if providers are unable to find a test they are looking for, they are more likely to create a write-in order, whether in CPOE (if permitted) or using a manual requisition.[15] CPOE systems may decrease write-in orders because CPOE provides the opportunity to display a larger test menu, reducing the need for handwritten orders.[15]

Ordering Messages and Alerts

Most CPOE systems support the display of test-specific ordering messages that can be used to improve order quality and reduce inappropriate or incorrect ordering.[16] Alert messages may be designed as "interruptive" or "noninterruptive." Noninterruptive alerts passively display test information and ordering advice, and do not require a specific acknowledgment or response by the ordering clinician. An example of an effective noninterruptive alert was shown in a study implementing a CPOE alert for the 1,25-(OH)$_2$ vitamin D test, directing clinicians to order 25-OH vitamin D (the appropriate test for routine screening) instead.[17] This alert message improved order correctness with a greater than 70% decline in inappropriate orders for 1,25-(OH)$_2$ vitamin D. Other information that may be useful to display to reduce inappropriate ordering may include test turnaround time, prior and pending test results, performing laboratory, and test cost.[18-21]

Noninterruptive alerts are a valuable tool to provide key information to clinicians without placing a substantial burden in terms of lost time or workflow impact[22]; however, the downside of this passive approach is that noninterruptive alerts can be inadvertently overlooked or deliberately ignored. Moreover, in many CPOE systems, the "help text" for a given order is not visible without the user navigating to another screen, and therefore noninterruptive alerts may have more limited utility in these settings. Interruptive alerts, in contrast, intentionally create a pause in the workflow by requiring acknowledgment or the provision of further information before an order can be finalized. Most often taking the form of "pop-up" boxes, interruptive alerts may be less likely to be inadvertently overlooked and can be effective when used judiciously.

Interruptive alerts can be used to educate providers about important changes in practice that may impact clinical care. A recent study demonstrated the effectiveness of an interruptive alert in standardizing care (Figure 5-1).[23] The hospital in the study established a policy restricting the use of creatine kinase-MB (CK-MB) solely to patients that had recently undergone percutaneous coronary intervention. This was a significant change in process because the test had been included previously in the standard protocol for ruling out myocardial infarction. In addition to order set changes, the protocol was communicated in the CPOE system through an interruptive alert requiring the provider to enter the testing indication when attempting to order CK-MB. The captured indications were then audited by the laboratory, with emails sent to clinicians continuing to place inappropriate orders. This approach resulted in a sustained reduction in CK-MB testing of approximately 80%, and the residual testing was deemed to be clinically appropriate.

A key consideration when designing alerting strategies is *alert fatigue*.[24] Alert fatigue is a phenomenon whereby clinicians are overwhelmed with alert messages and begin ignoring alerts, which can create significant patient safety concerns because highly important alerts may be ignored along with less relevant ones. Because alert fatigue may reduce the general effectiveness of all alerts, even those that may be well designed or relevant, it is important to design alerts with the risk of alert fatigue in mind. Strategies to reduce alert fatigue may include limiting the number of alerts, reserving interruptive alerts for the most important situations, and making alerts as clear, concise, and relevant as possible. Periodic monitoring of alert effectiveness should be a mandatory component of any interruptive alert system, with ineffective alerts removed or redesigned.[25]

CPOE Order Sets

Electronic ordering templates (ie, order sets) are typically created for specific clinical situations or circumstances, such as the inpatient management of community-acquired pneumonia. Templates may include orders for nursing, medications, laboratory tests, and radiology studies. For example, a community-acquired pneumonia template may include not only antibiotic and x-ray orders, but also orders for complete blood cell counts and blood cultures. Templates may positively impact patient safety because clinicians will be guided to select from the tests contained on the template, which, in a well-designed template, will be appropriate for most clinical scenarios.[26] Templates may help prevent needed tests from being overlooked. Several studies have demonstrated how incorporation of clinical practice guidelines into templates or other CPOE ordering screens may improve test or blood product utilization.[17,27,28]

Poorly designed order sets can negatively impact patient safety and the quality of care because errors or omissions in a template can potentially affect every patient for which the template is used. Thus, the development and maintenance of CPOE order sets needs to be a carefully controlled process.[29,30] Before use, a review of each order set should be carried out by a committee with representation of all disciplines included in the order set (eg, pharmacy, radiology, laboratory, nursing). Each order set should have an assigned owner responsible for the clinical content and should be periodically monitored for content and usage. In addition, the knowledge management system should have utilities to facilitate the identification of outdated tests or medications in order sets. Usability considerations with order sets are essential because CPOE order sets are often logistically much more challenging to fill out than the paper forms they replace.[29]

Corollary Orders

An additional way that CPOE systems can facilitate patient safety is with the use of corollary order notifications.[31] *Corollary laboratory orders* (also known as *consequent orders*) are orders for laboratory tests that are required or recommended as a result of other orders. For example, patients receiving intravenous heparin require monitoring of the partial thromboplastin time (PTT) to assess the level of anticoagulation and require regular platelet counts to screen for heparin-induced thrombocytopenia. Many CPOE systems have the functionality to remind clinicians to enter these corollary orders at the time of the initial heparin order.

CPOE Search and Screen Modifications

It is well established that modifying CPOE order screens and test search parameters may have important effects on utilization.[15,32-36] In addition, these changes can also have patient safety implications

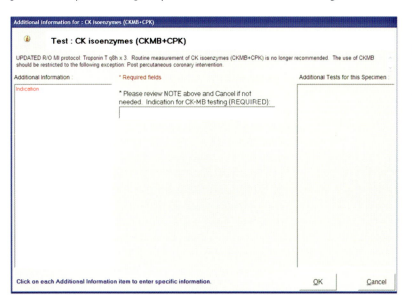

Figure 5-1. Example of an interruptive laboratory alert for creatine kinase-MB (CK-MB). Clinicians attempting to order CK-MB are presented with the interruptive alert screen as shown. The alert requires that the user enter an indication for testing or cancel the testing.

because needed tests may be omitted if not found easily. For example, including *celiac* as a search term for tests including anti–tissue transglutaminase IgA and anti–gliadin IgA can assist clinicians in finding the appropriate test, even if they lack knowledge of the test's name. Conversely, omitting search terms, making tests more difficult to find, can lead to incorrect tests being ordered or delays in diagnosis.

CPOE Implementation

One of the highest periods of patient safety risk with CPOE systems is during the implementation phase.[37] CPOE systems are typically a component of the larger electronic health record (EHR). In some EHR systems, the LIS is a module within the greater EHR system.[38] In these systems, there may be less integration risk because the CPOE module and laboratory module are components of the same system and there is a single vendor involved. In other instances, the CPOE system and the LIS will be products from different vendors and thus will need to electronically communicate via a custom interface. This is an area of patient risk because of nonstandard interfacing protocols and the complexity of the relationship of the EHR to the laboratory system. In all scenarios, the complexity of the ordering and reporting interfaces requires large investments in planning and testing during implementation.

The initial phases of a CPOE project are often critical to success because poorly designed orders and interfaces may be challenging to incrementally fix once established due to the fact that individual test orders serve as the building blocks used to construct order sets, provider preference lists, and decision support rules. Having a thoughtful, complete set of tests early in the process allows these higher order functions to move ahead to create care pathways that can improve patient safety and prevent errors.

Patient safety risks occur when systems are inadequately tested before going live.[39,40] Before any actual testing, it is essential that all workflows are clearly documented and a highly detailed testing plan is developed. Areas of patient safety concerns during CPOE implementations include canceled orders, duplicate tests, specimen sources, and order comments. It is important that all CPOE orders undergo comprehensive testing, with each possible CPOE test being ordered, resulted in the laboratory system, and results reviewed in all available EHR result displays to ensure all result components are properly displayed. Attention to test-naming conventions, abbreviations, and synonyms are important because the search results and test display names are major factors in test selection.[15]

Clinical Decision Support

CDS systems are now a part of most EHR systems and often incorporate laboratory testing in their rules-based approaches.[41] Analogous systems for medication ordering have been shown to significantly decrease adverse drug events and are now widely implemented in CPOE systems.[33,42] Similar approaches can further improve test ordering by suggesting additional tests for consideration, recommending more appropriate assays, or warning of the presence of a medication or clinical condition that may interfere with test interpretation. Furthermore, whereas many current CDS systems attempt to replicate advice or knowledge that an expert clinician would provide, future systems may serve to provide information that is distinct from that which the human brain can produce. For example, modern statistical and computational algorithms may be able to identify subtle patterns in large data sets that would be inaccessible to the human brain but that can inform diagnosis or clinical management.[43,44] Statistical approaches have also been applied to laboratory error detection and may in the future help to improve laboratory quality management and resource utilization.[45]

Specimen Collection

Laboratory CPOE is an enabler for the deployment of specimen collection systems that may be used to improve the accuracy of patient identification and patient safety. The specimen collection systems may be a part of the EHR, the LIS, or a third-party system. The key parts to the system are typically software and handheld devices that retrieve active orders from the LIS and enable bedside label printing and specimen labeling only after scanning a patient's barcoded wristband. These systems also capture the actual collection time and phlebotomist identification, and can send this information to the LIS. This "just-in-time" model can largely eliminate specimen mislabeling if proper procedures are followed. In addition, labels generated from the laboratory system indicate the required tube type, providing additional decision support at the bedside. Bedside labeling systems have been shown to reduce labeling and wrong-tube errors in both inpatient and emergency room settings.[46-50]

Outpatient specimen collection can be problematic with respect to specimen labeling because of the lack of patient wristbands or other forms of electronically verifiable identification in most outpatient settings. With outpatient CPOE systems, electronic orders may be present, but the process of creating barcoded specimen labels does not have the same electronic check that can be implemented for inpatient specimens. Moreover, outpatient care facilities and specimen collection processes are complex, and specimen label printers may not be co-located near the point of collection for logistical, technical, or financial reasons; in these cases, there are patient safety risks created by requiring the specimen to be relabeled or having the labels printed at a location distant from the patient. These risks can be minimized by the thoughtful location of specimen label printers, awareness of the risks, and processes put in place to mitigate risk.

Collection Instructions

An additional source of preanalytic error is tests that are not collected or processed properly.[1] An example would be patients failing to have trough antibiotic levels drawn per protocol (eg, before the third dose) or lactate tests not placed on ice after collection. These types of errors can lead to erroneous test results. In some situations, technology has increased the opportunity for these patient safety gaps because these types of special instructions were traditionally written on paper requisitions seen by the person collecting the specimen and by laboratory personnel. With electronic order entry systems, care needs to be taken to ensure that these test instructions are still brought to the attention of the person collecting the specimen. This can be accomplished by ensuring collection instructions are viewable on the handheld devices used for specimen collection and/or printed on specimen labels. In addition to collection instructions specific to the test, provider instructions entered during the order (eg, "swab left knee wound") must also be brought to the attention of the person collecting the specimen. This may require transmission of these instructions to the LIS in a manner such that the instructions will be viewable during the collection process.

Other patient safety concerns may occur with the collection of stat and timed specimens. For stat specimens, if there is a significant difference between stat and routine processing times, it will be important that stat specimens are clearly differentiated from the routine specimens so that errors and delays in care do not result. The designation of a stat order in the CPOE system must be transmitted to the LIS and prompt changes to the collection and handling processes for the specimen. In timed orders (eg, therapeutic drug levels, including many antibiotics, immunosuppressive medications, and antiepileptic drugs), the accurate timing of specimen collection is essential for result interpretation.[51] Failure to collect the specimen at the designated time can lead to inappropriate dosing adjustments, inaccurate assessment of toxicity, and unnecessary follow-up tests. Decision support that links timed drug monitoring orders to medication doses has been proposed as a solution to these errors.[52,53]

Order Provider Identification

In CPOE, the identity of the ordering provider is another common source of patient safety concerns. There may be several providers for a given test order: the attending provider, the ordering provider, the encounter provider, and the billing provider. In the simplest case of a patient seen directly by his or her primary care physician, this clinician may assume all four of these roles. However, in the team-based care that is becoming more common, the patient could be seen by a nurse practitioner and a resident, with the attending provider retaining responsibility for test follow-up. In these situations, it is important that the laboratory and EHR interfaces be constructed properly to provide the laboratory with the information needed to complete all necessary tasks, including billing, routine-result reporting, and critical value reporting.

Specimen Processing

Upon reaching the laboratory, there are several points in the processing pathway where technology can reduce the risks to patient safety.[54-56] Automated processing equipment that can centrifuge, uncap, decant, and aliquot specimens into automatically labeled daughter tubes eliminates the inherently risky step of manual decanting and relabeling, with its attendant errors in specimen identification. In addition, add-on test processes are an area of high risk because tests can mistakenly be added onto an inappropriate specimen, an outdated specimen, or the wrong patient's specimen. Several automation systems feature specimen "stockyards" that can retain unused specimen tubes, and, after entering the add-on test in the laboratory system, the system can automatically retrieve the tube and place it back on the automation line for additional testing.

Analytic Phase

Instrumentation

Modern instrumentation and automation have reduced many opportunities for errors and patient safety issues during the analytic phase (Table 5-2).[54,57,58] Automated serum indices for lipemia, icterus, and hemolysis can reliably identify specimens with potential interferences, and these specimens can be rejected or annotated to prevent inaccurately filed results.[59] In addition, instruments that can automatically detect and flag samples with bubbles, clots, insufficient sample volume, or other unsuitable characteristics are important for the reduction of analytic error. The use of these technologies has become increasingly important to patient safety in highly automated laboratories, where visual inspection of the tube may not be possible or practical.

Laboratory Information System

The LIS is the system responsible for laboratory data management and plays a critical role coordinating laboratory workflow.[60] LIS deployment should support the following patient safety goals: (1) avoid manual, error-prone processes; (2) detect errors that do occur; (3) improve workflow and productivity; and (4) provide clinicians with timely, interpretable results. The avoidance of manual processes should be a central element of every LIS implementation. Instrument interfaces, carefully designed autoverification, and heavy utilization of barcodes for specimen identification and tracking have all been proven to reduce errors within the laboratory.[61,62] Moreover, the standardization of interfaces and terminologies has led to the integration of the LIS into the health care information network. Interfaces for orders (via CPOE), demographics (via registration systems), and results can improve the accuracy and timeliness of the entire laboratory testing process. Achieving the goal of a highly connected, shareable EHR requires the increasingly tight connection of the LIS to the rest of the health care system.

Specimen Identification and Barcoding

Manual laboratory data entry is an important source of laboratory error, with manual entry processes demonstrated to produce average error rates of 2.8%.[63] Transpositions of digits or misplaced decimal places are especially difficult to detect and can lead to incorrect results being reported, with patient safety implications. CPOE with electronic transmission of orders from the CPOE system to the LIS is an important strategy for reducing manual transcription and its attendant errors. In addition, barcodes are heavily utilized in the laboratory to identify and track specimens throughout the testing process.[62,64] In most systems, each tube of a specimen is uniquely identified with a barcode. For tube identification, laboratories typically use linear or one-dimensional barcodes (a series of black lines and spaces). The linear barcode on a laboratory specimen label typically encodes the container identifier (CID), which is the unique identifier for the specimen container. Formats for the linear barcodes used in laboratories include Code 39 and Code 128. A major limitation of linear barcodes is that they can practically contain only very limited information, with less than a dozen characters able to fit on a typically sized tube label. Two-dimensional (2D) barcode formats, such as PDF417 and Data Matrix, store data using two dimensions of a surface. This enables more data to be represented in the barcode, with some 2D formats holding hundreds of characters in 1 cm². The major disadvantage of the 2D barcodes is that they need a more sophisticated barcode reader than the simple readers used for linear barcodes. Barcode specimen labels allow simplified specimen tracking throughout the laboratory with the use of automated barcode scanners or manual scanning by laboratory staff. Most highly automated instruments will have barcode scanners incorporated into the instrument to permit automatic identification and tracking of barcoded specimens.

Radio-frequency identification (RFID) is an autoidentification technology that uses radio waves to identify objects. RFID systems use a small electronic tag that is read by an RFID scanner, analogous to the way that a barcode scanner reads a printed barcode. The RFID tag consists of a small, integrated circuit

Table 5-2. Technology for Patient Safety in the Analytic Phase	
Patient Safety Issue	**Technology Solution(s)**
Undetected analyzer problems (eg, clots, bubbles, hemolysis)	• Automated clot and bubble detection • Automated serum indices for hemolysis, icterus, lipemia • Delta checks • Patient moving averages
Patient identification errors	• Specimen barcodes • Robotic automation to reduce manual steps • Delta checks (simple or combinatorial)
Delays in sample processing	• CPOE with order communication • Bidirectional instrument interfaces • Automated monitoring and display of pending tests
Missed tests	• CPOE with order communication • Bidirectional instrument interfaces • Reflex testing protocols
Resulting errors	• Bidirectional instrument interfaces • Autovalidation rules to prevent accidental release of inaccurate data
Dilution errors	• Automated dilutions controlled by instruments or middleware

CPOE, computerized provider order entry.

attached to an antenna. Data related to the tagged object are stored in the memory of the integrated circuit. Information is sent wirelessly to or from the RFID tag via radio-frequency signals generated by the RFID scanner. RFID tags can hold large amounts of information, can be very rugged, and can be read through other materials, not requiring a line of sight between the reader and tag. Furthermore, an RFID reader can scan multiple RFID tags simultaneously, in contrast to the barcode process, in which each barcoded item must be individually oriented before scanning. RFID tags may be well suited for numerous applications in the laboratory testing process, including specimen tracking and patient wristband identification. The current limitations of RFID include the cost of tags and readers, as well as the need for additional infrastructure and middleware to be able to utilize the tag data in laboratory information systems.

Manual Results Entry

Numerous laboratory assays are performed on instruments that are either not capable of being interfaced (eg, viscometers) or that may be used too infrequently to have interfacing be financially viable. For low-volume testing platforms, LIS interfaces can be costly—in terms of both the capital and the labor—to install and validate the interface. For testing performed on noninterfaced instruments, the LIS typically provides a printed worksheet of pending orders organized with blank space to permit manual result transcription and to facilitate subsequent manual result entry in the LIS. Given the high rate of transcription errors due to keystroke mistakes, it is essential to have a quality assurance plan in place to oversee manual resulting. The use of automated delta checks or range checks can assist in error prevention in these settings. In addition, the use of specimen barcodes throughout the manual testing process can help to prevent specimen identification errors.

Instrument Interfaces

Most laboratory tests are performed on analyzers that exchange data with the LIS through instrument interfaces. Interfacing high-volume automated instruments with the LIS greatly improves productivity and reduces opportunities for error. Instrument interfaces can be unidirectional or bidirectional. Unidirectional interfaces typically send results from the analyzer to the LIS. In a unidirectional interface, no data are transmitted from the LIS to the instrument, so orders and patient/specimen identifying information must be entered into the analyzer, providing an opportunity for ordering errors to occur. The unique CID for each tube of the specimen can serve as the identifying link in these scenarios because the CID in the LIS is associated with the patient demographics. In addition, because the CID is typically barcoded on the specimen tube, having the analyzer scan the tube's barcode can provide a simple way to provide specimen-identifying information to the analyzer.

A bidirectional interface permits the LIS and analyzer to send data back and forth, eliminating the need for the direct entry of orders and patient/specimen identifiers in the analyzer, and thus eliminating a key source of error. Bidirectional interfaces are essentially required for analyzers (such as chemistry systems) where a wide variety of different tests may be performed on a given sample. With a bidirectional interface, the LIS sends patient/specimen identifiers and orders to the analyzer, and the analyzer sends the results back to the LIS. If the laboratory is already entering orders into the LIS, a bidirectional interface eliminates the need for reentering orders and patient/specimen identifiers in the analyzer.

The LIS and Quality Assurance

The LIS is essential to the laboratory for quality assurance. The LIS provides the data elements necessary for the monitoring of assay turnaround time because it timestamps the key events for a laboratory test, including order time, collection time, accessioning time (ie, the time that each order is entered into the LIS), in-laboratory receipt time, and result time. Specimens that have been received by the LIS but not yet resulted will appear on the technologist's pending test list. Specimens that have remained on the pending test list for longer than the usual periods of time may need to be investigated. Technology to automatically run pending reports and display key performance metrics, especially delayed results, on monitors throughout the laboratory may provide enhanced attention to delayed results and improve turnaround time.

In addition to turnaround time reports, a wide variety of other management reports are available from the LIS, including testing volumes, workload statistics, and billing reports. In addition, the ability to create ad hoc reports from the LIS is supported in most laboratory information systems. A sample ad hoc report would be to "retrieve the phlebotomy locations of all hemolyzed specimens." The LIS should provide views and reporting tools, such that the LIS staff of an organization can easily create reports to ask important management and patient safety questions.[65]

Results Review

The validation of results is an important function of the LIS. The initial result of an assay is typically flagged as "prelim," awaiting review by a technologist. The LIS then provides an interface where technologists can review and release (ie, finalize) results. Many of the rules and calculations necessary for result reporting reside in the LIS. Calculations of the international normalized ratio (INR), the anion gap, and the estimated glomerular filtration rate are examples of simple calculations performed by the LIS. It is essential that the laboratory carefully test calculations, especially in situations involving unknown patient age, out-of-range results, and corrected results.

To ensure that only valid results are released, the LIS may apply rules to the result to compare the test result with the reportable range for the analyte, the reference range, and the critical value limits. In addition, the current result may be compared to the patient's prior results (a delta check) to alert the technologist to possible erroneous results.[66] Large changes in results over short time intervals are more likely to be erroneous results. Most LISs are able to incorporate delta check rules into result-reporting processes such that a sample failing a delta check is reviewed for accuracy before release to the medical record. For certain analytes, however, the delta check may not provide sufficient sensitivity and specificity to be useful.[67] In the example of inpatient creatinine testing, a simple delta check rule was shown to have only fair sensitivity and specificity to identify patients with a rising creatinine indicative of acute kidney injury.[68] In the case of creatinine, the comparison of the patient's current value to the 72-hour patient minimum value improved the laboratory's ability to identify patients at risk for acute kidney injury.[68] Implementation of such calculations within the LIS can provide a means to flag results and alert clinicians of impending patient safety concerns. Another example of an enhancement to the standard one-parameter delta check was shown for complete blood cell (CBC) count results, where the combination of delta checks from selected CBC count parameters was demonstrated to improve the sensitivity and specificity for detecting patient identification errors and other specimen-related errors.[69]

Autoverification

Traditional technologist result verification relies on "mental algorithms" that are applied to single results or groups of results. Reliance on individual judgment can lead to variability in processes and error. Autoverification (automatic verification) refers to the process where computer-based algorithms perform actions on laboratory results without review by a technologist.[61] The actions performed may include results release, dilution and retesting, order cancellation, repeat analysis, reflexive testing, or result comment addition. Most commonly, autoverification algorithms are used to automatically release results without the need for technologist review. To facilitate autoverification, most LISs have a parameter, the *release range*, that can be defined for each test for the purpose of autoverification. A carefully designed autoverification algorithm can lead to improved turnaround times, increased operational efficiency, and a more consistent process.[61,70] Autoverification rules may reside in the LIS or in middleware (see below). In order for autoverification to be implemented safely, the characteristics of the test must be thoroughly understood and validated. A typical autoverification rule would permit test values for a particular analyte to be autoreleased provided the resulted value falls within a specified autoverification range (ie, the release range), no quality control failures are present, and no instrument flags are present. Delta checks are also commonly incorporated into autoverification algorithms. Autoverification algorithms should be thoroughly tested and periodically reevaluated to ensure that the rules are performing as expected.

Middleware

In addition to test results, decisions during the analytic phase of laboratory testing may depend on unreported test parameters, additional analyzer data, quality assurance/quality control data, and the results of other tests, as well as historical test performance data. Many current LISs do not have access to this data, let alone have the capacity to generate an integrated display of such disparate information or to incorporate these data elements into rules and algorithms. To address this need, laboratory *middleware* (software in the "middle" between the LIS and the laboratory instruments) has been developed to extend the capabilities of the traditional LIS. Middleware may be supplied by the instrument vendor or a third party and provides an environment for sophisticated rules-based processing. In addition to providing integrated data displays, middleware can support more sophisticated rules-based logic and centralized control of instrumentation. Middleware can improve patient safety by rapidly performing a large number of checks on the sample before permitting the results to be finalized. Middleware can also use approaches such as the calculation and analysis of patient moving averages to elucidate shifts and trends indicative of quality issues in the testing system. The more advanced rule-based approaches, available through middleware and some advanced LISs, allow rules to be authored that can provide control of retesting, alert when interfering conditions are present, and permit reflex testing across multiple specimens and instruments, as well as support automated test add-ons and specimen tracking.

Table 5-3. Technology for Patient Safety in the Postanalytic Phase	
Patient Safety Issue	**Technology Solution(s)**
Result transmission problems	• Active monitoring of interfaces and error queues
Result trends not noticed by provider	• Laboratory information system (LIS) or middleware flagging of results due to delta check failures • LIS or middleware flagging of results due to change from patient's baseline value
Critical value reporting delays	• Use of LIS functionality to provide an interruptive alert to laboratory staff when critical values are resulted • Automated provider critical value notification • Systems to track and maintain the responding provider for critical results • Centralized customer service centers to make critical result calls
Missed follow-up for tests pending at discharge	• Centralized reporting of test results post discharge • Routing of postdischarge results to a designated provider's result management system
Errors during manual entry of laboratory results in the electronic health record (EHR)	• Limit result entry whenever possible with direct interfaces • Limit user access to result entry functionality in EHR • Enhance data entry screens to minimize opportunities for errors • Clearly identify the result as externally entered (eg, with use of "EXTERNAL" as a prefix to the test name)
Misinterpretation of laboratory test results	• Comments attached to test results • Infobuttons to link online test information to test results • Pathologist-created narrative interpretations
Errors and delays in the reporting of reference laboratory test results	• Bidirectional interfaces with reference laboratories

Reflex Testing Protocols

Reflex testing protocols allow for additional tests to be ordered depending on the results of the first test or tests. In addition to their documented impact on utilization management, reflex protocols can improve patient safety by preventing errors and missed follow-up tests during laboratory testing workups.[71] Thyroid test algorithms are an example of a common reflex protocol. Most algorithms start with the thyroid stimulating hormone (TSH) test: if the TSH is normal, then no further testing is performed; however, an abnormal TSH is automatically followed up with additional studies as required to work up the abnormal TSH result and to provide additional diagnostic information. In addition to preventing errors, the appropriate use of reflex testing may reduce unnecessary testing. Although CPOE systems are not required to establish reflex protocols, CPOE systems make it practical to offer a large menu of clinically appropriate reflex testing panels because providers can search for tests and panels.

Postanalytic Phase

Interfaces to the Electronic Health Record

After finalization, laboratory results are typically sent via electronic interfaces to the EHR. This step is generally transparent to the end user in the laboratory but is an area where patient safety concerns may arise due to problems with the transmission of some or all of the results. In many health care systems there are often several "stops" a laboratory result takes before being posted in the medical record (Table 5-3). The software and systems that control the routing of result messages are termed *interface engines*. The presence and complexity of many interface engines provide novel opportunities for transmission failure. Having monitoring tools in place to rapidly identify and correct transmission failures is essential to avoid delayed EHR reporting, which can compromise patient safety. Transmission failures may be total (eg, all laboratory results not transmitting), module specific (eg, microbiology results not posting), test specific (eg, due to an order code mapping issue), or sporadic (eg, issues with patients with long last names). All of these possibilities should be monitored with a combination of active interface monitoring and error queue checking.

Result Review

The postanalytic phase of testing involves result access and interpretation by clinicians. Failure to review and follow up on outpatient test results represents a common patient safety and malpractice concern.[72,73] EHRs generally provide tools for test result management, but the creation of policies, expectations, and monitoring of test result follow-up is needed at the institutional level to ensure patient safety. Optimal reporting relies not only on data availability, but on a presentation that makes result interpretation intuitive, efficient, and unambiguous. Well-designed electronic reporting applications can improve retrieval efficiency and clarity by highlighting recent results, grouping related tests, and enabling clinicians to filter results based on time intervals. Moreover, the availability of customizable, user-friendly charts and graphs allow identification of time-based patterns and inter-test relationships. The laboratory does not typically control data display within results viewers such as the hospital's EHR system, patient portals, or mobile-format results viewers; however, laboratory accreditation requirements require that the laboratory validate the display of laboratory results in downstream result-viewing applications.[10,11,74] The validation of laboratory results display should pay particular attention to the appearance of result flagging, reference intervals, specimen comments, reporting-laboratory location, columnar data, long text comments, and corrected results. The laboratory must work collaboratively with the hospital EHR group to ensure that laboratory data are properly formatted and presented for maximal clinical efficiency and safety. In addition, the laboratory must ensure that the format and content of results printed from the EHR and other applications (including the LIS itself) meet all regulatory requirements for printed laboratory reports.

Critical Value Reporting

The reporting of laboratory results that require urgent clinical review was originally highlighted in the 1970s by Lundberg, who defined a laboratory result as critical if it suggested imminent danger to a patient unless appropriate action was promptly initiated.[75] Since this initial description, hospitals and laboratories worldwide have adopted the practice of identifying and reporting such laboratory results in a systematic manner. Errors or delays in reporting results that require urgent clinical review can have serious patient care and medicolegal consequences. Thus, reporting systems need to be carefully designed and monitored to ensure patient safety and maximize efficient communication. The reliability of critical value reporting is an important measure of laboratory quality because it contributes significantly to clinical effectiveness, patient safety, and operational efficiency.

Critical value limits are defined in the LIS test dictionary. An example of a critical value would be a potassium result of 8.0 mEq/L. Such a patient with severe hyperkalemia would be at risk of potentially fatal abnormal heart rhythms. It is imperative that the LIS rapidly alerts a laboratory technologist to a critical value because the patient's care team needs to be contacted without delay. Many LISs have functionality that can provide automatic and interruptive alerts to laboratory staff for critical values and allow the documentation of the subsequent communication to the care team. These systems can improve patient safety by enabling critical values to be more promptly addressed. In addition, the centralization of callback using a callback module can improve safety by allowing critical callbacks to be performed by customer service call centers, the use of which were recently highlighted as an evidence-based best practice.[76] Furthermore, reports generated from LIS callback systems can simplify the monitoring of key callback metrics and permit follow-up for outliers.

Flagging of Abnormal/Critical Results

The ability of the LIS to flag a test result as critical or abnormal and to pass that flag along to the EHR is important to enable downstream notification systems. In many EHR systems, flagged results are handled differently in the results management module of the EHR. For example, some EHRs are able to both highlight and require active acknowledgment for results flagged as critical. Moreover, the EHR may facilitate the linkage of acknowledgment to action taken. This can be accomplished within the EHR via functionality that permits the provider acknowledging the result to act on the result, for example, to order a follow-up test, order a medication, create a referral to a specialist, or notify the patient.

For tests with numeric results, LIS dictionaries typically have test level parameters that may be specified to define the alert thresholds for each test. In addition, many LISs are able to implement rules to create an alert only for the first time in a specified time interval that the critical result occurs (eg, alert for low platelet count only once per 24 hours) or permit different alert thresholds for different patient locations. In addition, other calculations can be used to compare the current result with the prior result and to set a result flag when a certain difference is present (ie, a delta check flag). Alert thresholds may also be set with respect to patient age, gender, and setting. Utilization of the full rules-based capabilities of the LIS to flag results can provide a highly customized and laboratory-specific set of alerts. Results of qualitative tests, such as microbiology cultures, may not have critical or abnormal flags attached to them because of limitations within the LIS as well as the challenge in defining the normal range for some nonnumeric tests. The lack of microbiology flagging can create patient safety issues in the EHR because the presence of a flag is often used as the basis for filtering results and alerts clinicians to look more closely at a given result. In some circumstances, custom interface or LIS work may be necessary to enable flagging of abnormal or critical microbiology results. Dependence on the LIS to flag critical results mandates a careful approach during LIS downtimes when testing may occur without the presence of the LIS. The manual procedures used by the laboratory during LIS downtimes should ensure that critical results are appropriately recognized and communicated.

Automated Reporting Systems for Critical Values

Given the high volume and potentially error-prone nature of verbal communications, automation of the critical callback process would seem to be highly desirable. In addition to potential improvements in the timeliness of communication, the removal of this responsibility from frontline laboratory staff could lead to a reduction in stress for the laboratory and permit the laboratory to focus on other tasks. Reliable identification of an available, responding provider must be the cornerstone of any automated approach. Additional key elements required for successful implementation of an automated critical value reporting system include the following: (1) a reliable paging, Short Messaging Service (SMS), or other messaging system; (2) a method to permit active acknowledgment by the responsible caregiver; (3) a robust escalation procedure when acknowledgment does not occur within a specified time frame; and (4) downtime procedures. In general, the LIS is not able to directly interact with paging or SMS systems. Therefore, middleware or custom solutions are often used to implement automated notification systems. If patient results are to be provided in the automated messages, privacy and security should be considered because there is a risk that patient data may be transmitted via nonsecure communications or may be stored on devices lacking encryption. In addition, downstream devices should be validated to ensure accurate presentation of the entire results message (including patient identifiers) and all result data, including test name, value, units, reference interval, flags, collection time, and result comments.

Several studies have demonstrated improvements in the timeliness of critical result reporting with the use of a variety of automated notification systems.[76-80] However, a 2012 systematic review of the literature regarding automation of inpatient critical result notification concluded that there was insufficient evidence to fully endorse the automation of inpatient result communication as a laboratory medicine best practice.[76] If automation of critical result reporting is considered, it is important for laboratories to not only examine the timeliness of communication, but also to examine the system's impact on the action taken after communication of the result. For example, an automatic page to the two-way alphanumeric paging device of the requesting provider may satisfy regulatory requirements for communication to the provider, but unless that provider reliably communicates the result to the clinical team that can take action, the clinical benefit of the rapid communication may not be present. Regardless of the method used to automate communication, it is essential that the entire communication process be examined to ensure that the implemented system leads to the desired outcomes.

Responsible Provider Systems

A key building block of a high-reliability, critical result reporting process is the reliable identification of the provider who can and should take action on a critical test result.[81] CPOE systems with electronic order communication can aid in the high-reliability transmission of results to the responsible caregiver; however, in many situations, the provider ordering the test may not be the appropriate person to respond to the critical result. In acute care settings, the provider with responsibility for a patient's results may change at each shift, and it may not be clear which caregiver is responsible during care transitions. In addition, in many clinical settings, team-based approaches to patient care are being increasingly implemented, and test result triage and management may be performed by members of the care team besides the provider requesting the test. A potential solution to this issue is the creation of the distinct role of the "responsible caregiver" for each patient, a single person who should be notified with an urgent clinical issue such as a critical value.[81] The downside of this approach is that for the identification of the responsible caregiver to be accurate, it requires continuous updating of the responsible caregiver role.

Tests Pending at Discharge

Patients are often discharged from hospital inpatient stays and emergency room visits before all laboratory tests are completed.[82] A number of studies have demonstrated that providers are often unaware of tests resulted after discharge, and that follow-up for abnormal tests resulted post discharge is poor.[83-85] The reasons for this poor performance include lack of mechanisms to track these tests and unclear responsibility for follow-up.[81] In recognition of this patient safety concern, in many institutions these results are triaged to a central person or a designated person on the care team to assure follow-up with the patient and relevant providers. For example, EHR test result routing rules can deliver all inpatient results occurring post discharge to the electronic mailbox of the inpatient attending who most recently oversaw the care of the patient.

Infobuttons

With the increasing number of test options and complexity, many clinicians are unable to maintain sufficient knowledge to correctly interpret complex test results in all clinical circumstances. The provision of relevant, context-specific clinical information at the time of clinical decision making is the goal of just-in-time knowledge management.[86] Several groups have demonstrated the automated retrieval of context-specific information from network-accessible resources, guided by contextual data extracted from clinical applications.[87-89] In each of these examples, a resource management system (called the InfoButton Manager by one group) sits in-between the clinical application and the network resources. The InfoButton Manager receives contextual information from a clinical application and matches this to the appropriate resources. In this manner, a single mouse click can provide context-relevant laboratory testing reference materials, Medline references, locally produced clinical practice guidelines, and articles from subscription-based resources, all of which can be brought to bear on the clinical question. For example, a clinician reviewing results for anemia testing can, with a single click, obtain several recent review articles, a locally created diagnostic algorithm for anemia, and information regarding testing options for anemia in the hospital laboratory.

Result Interpretation

Rules can be implemented in the LIS to attach coded comments (short interpretive paragraphs) to provide interpretive support for complex test results. For example, hepatitis B test panel results may be accompanied by an automatically generated coded comment that can differ based on the results of the hepatitis panel. The quality and utility of these "canned comments" varies widely, and the effectiveness of these approaches is unclear.[90-93] In recent years, there has been interest in pathologist-provided interpretive reporting for complex laboratory evaluations such as coagulation and immunology workups.[94] In this approach, a pathologist expert reviews the laboratory testing in the context of the patient's clinical condition and creates a patient-specific interpretive report that is transmitted to the medical record and is available alongside the test results. Interpretive laboratory reports may include a narrative describing the differential diagnosis, pertinent details about the assays that may affect their interpretation, and suggestions for additional testing. Narrative interpretations created by clinical pathology experts appear to provide positive benefits to the physician, the patient, and the hospital.[95]

Reference Laboratory Testing

Testing performed at outside reference laboratories can introduce patient safety risks due to the differences in logistics and reporting that may be present for reference laboratory testing versus on-site testing. Reference laboratory tests in many cases are not electronically interfaced, and the ordering and resulting of these tests may require manual processes. Another item to be considered is that many reference laboratory tests may be performed infrequently or have long analytic times, and thus the turnaround time for these results may be measured in weeks, complicating result tracking.

Many reference laboratories are capable of being electronically interfaced using a standard (Health Level Seven International [HL7]) interface implemented securely via options such as a virtual private network (VPN). The interfaces are generally between the sending hospital LIS and the reference laboratory LIS, but interfaces can also be set up directly between the EHR and the reference laboratory. Interfaces can be unidirectional or bidirectional. Unidirectional interfaces send the laboratory results back to the ordering facility LIS or EHR. With a unidirectional interface, there is no link to the test order. This type of interface is problematic when orders are generated electronically in the EHR because the reference laboratory results may not match up to the orders and CPOE orders may thus remain pending. In facilities with CPOE for laboratory orders, a bidirectional interface is generally used. In bidirectional interfaces, when orders are placed at the ordering facility, the LIS order is transmitted to the reference laboratory. For both types of interfaces there must be detailed mapping set up between the reference laboratory results and the result components of the sending facility LIS.

Certain reference laboratory results (eg, human immunodeficiency virus [HIV] phenotyping) are highly complex, and the result reports may include multicolor graphs and tables that are needed for optimal interpretation of the results. In many cases, the primary report format for these results is the Portable Document Format (PDF). PDF results can, in some cases, be sent via the electronic reference laboratory interface, but this requires that the reference laboratory LIS, the sending facility LIS, and the interfaces are all properly configured to handle PDF results. In addition, the viewing of PDF results in the EHR is variably supported. Health care systems should work with their EHR system, reference laboratories, and LIS to ensure that these complex results in their full report format (ie, PDF) are included in the medical record.

External Result Entry

Many EHRs permit authorized users to manually enter laboratory results into a patient's medical record. This is deemed necessary in many systems since patient laboratory testing may be performed at laboratories that do not electronically interface their data into the EHR and the data may be required for clinical care or meaningful use measures. With external result entry, risks to patient safety occur due to manual result entry introducing the potential for transcription errors or errors of omission in the result values, units, reference ranges, flagging, test comments, reporting laboratory, and other aspects of the test. External results, for both clinical and regulatory reasons, should include all the relevant fields from the external laboratory report, including the result value, reference interval, comments, and laboratory name/address. In addition, the manual result entry screens of the EHR should be carefully designed and configured to minimize the opportunity for error and data omissions. Further, due to the risks of manual entry, it must be made clear to a provider later reviewing external results that the results were entered manually (eg, by appending the prefix "EXTERNAL" to the test name) and therefore should be subject to enhanced scrutiny. Limiting the users permitted to perform manual data entry to trained users only in areas where the data is absolutely required for clinical care or meaningful use measures is another strategy to mitigate the risk of manual result entry.

Point-of-Care Testing Results

With the rapid growth of point-of-care testing (POCT), there is increasing interest in having POCT results available in the EHR.[96] POCT has been growing in scope and volume, and may present patient safety risks when not available in the medical record. For example, the result of a positive influenza point-of-care test may be important in treatment and diagnosis decisions, and if not available in structured form in the medical record, it may be missed. Ideally, POCT results should be available alongside all other laboratory results. It is important that POCT results are clearly designated as "Point of Care" because many point-of-care tests are not directly comparable to the central laboratory version of the test, and trending of these results together can result in misinterpretation.

In most settings, transmission of POCT results to the LIS is a requisite step for POCT result availability in the EHR. Transmission of results from the point-of-care devices to the LIS most often occurs via an intermediate data management system (a *data manager*) interfaced with the individual POCT devices. The data manager then transmits data to the LIS. Some data management systems also provide functionality that permits authorized users to result noninterfaced manual testing (eg, rapid flu antigen, stool occult blood) into the data manager, facilitating transmission of these results into the LIS and EHR. Functionality within some EHRs allows authorized users to directly input the results of POCT into the EHR. These instances with direct manual entry of POCT results by nonlaboratory staff are areas of high risk that need to be closely monitored. Users authorized to enter POCT results should undergo training for this activity, and the functionality should be streamlined as much as possible to minimize manual data entry and possibilities for error.

Point-of-care interfaces differ from other result-reporting interfaces because for POCT the interface must simultaneously order and result the testing. Recent standardization of the interfaces between POCT devices, data managers, and the LIS has improved the transmission of POCT results to the LIS.[96] In addition, this standardization has enabled the development of "vendor-neutral" data managers capable of interacting with a wide array of point-of-care devices from different manufacturers. This permits an organization to have a single interface between the data manager and the LIS to transfer a wide array of POCT results. When POCT is interfaced, it creates stringent requirements for the accuracy of operator and patient identification, because incorrectly captured data will likely lead to interface errors and delays in result reporting. The use of barcoded operator badges and patient wristbands to identify users and patients has been shown to reduce the errors that occur with manual data entry.[97] The standard methodology for transferring results from POCT devices to the LIS/EHR is the use of docking stations. This is a major workflow limitation for many point-of-care tests because until the device is docked, the results are not sent to the EHR. The recent emergence of point-of-care data devices that utilize wireless technologies to eliminate the need for docking and facilitate the real-time transfer of results to the medical record is expected to increase the timeliness and availability of POCT information in the EHR.

Metrics and Analytics

Systems for gathering and analyzing laboratory and other related data are of key importance in designing for patient safety and for use in safety improvement initiatives. For each test, it is helpful not only to trend turnaround times, but to also understand other parameters, such as the ordering provider and the indications for testing. For example, if there is substantial variation in the frequency with which a certain test is ordered across a group of clinicians from the same specialty and across substantially similar patient populations, it is likely that some clinicians are underordering the test or others are overordering it. Having the data and tools to identify improper test ordering, both in aggregate and at the level of the individual provider, can enable targeted efforts to improve the use of the testing.

In addition, given the increasing role of CPOE, it may be useful to track not only test orders, but also data describing various user interactions with the CPOE system. Analysis of CPOE user searches has proven valuable to improve the ability of clinicians to find and identify the appropriate tests for their patients.[15] Tracking detailed CPOE user interaction data may also be helpful in monitoring the effects of various CPOE alerts. For example, an alert designed to implement an institutional policy related to the ordering of CK-MB was monitored in a highly detailed fashion, which enabled tracking of how frequently individual clinicians searched for CK-MB, saw the alert messages, and then decided *not* to order the test. Using this analysis, the authors were able to demonstrate not only the effectiveness of the alert, but also to show that this alert was effective in providing both just-in-time advice and long-term education.[23]

Transfusion Medicine

Transfusion medicine presents unique patient safety concerns due to the high-risk activity of providing blood products to patients. Despite widespread improvements in systems and processes, serious mistransfusion errors are unacceptably frequent. In the United States, mistransfusion has consistently been a leading cause of death from transfusion.[98,99] At many centers, the bedside check to ensure the right blood product is being given to the right patient at the right time is performed largely without the aid of technology. Historically, the response to this error-prone process has been the implementation of the two-person verification requirement to improve the accuracy of identification and matching of the patient and blood product; however, this does not provide an actual margin of safety, as demonstrated by large-scale audits of actual transfusion practices. In one such report, the failure to match wristband identification with the blood product label was observed in 25% of transfusions.[100]

Research has demonstrated that the performance of repetitive task functions such as number matching is aided through the use of technology.[101] In addition, mistransfusion events typically result from *lapse errors* (slip-ups) rather than cognitive mistakes or deliberate processes failures.[102] Lapse errors are more likely to occur during repetitive tasks when individuals are distracted, rushed, or tired—conditions often found in the settings where blood products are administered. Machines are not generally susceptible to lapse errors, and thus the application of technology would be expected to improve transfusion safety. Software and systems to perform an electronic bedside check for blood products are available and can provide an additional margin of safety. These systems work analogously to bedside medication administration systems, by creating a unique identifier for each blood product and associating it with the patient. The patient-identifying information is available on the barcode label of the blood product, facilitating automated matching (by barcode scanning) of the patient's wristband and the blood product.

Pretransfusion Testing

Another patient safety risk in blood transfusion involves collection of the pretransfusion sample for type and screen testing. This sample determines the blood type that the patient will receive and is an essential part of blood transfusion safety. To improve the safety of these samples, blood banks require documentation of the person collecting the sample and the collection time; however, it has been demonstrated that, despite these safeguards, a significant percentage of type and screen samples are drawn on the wrong patient or labeled with incorrect patient identifiers. A solution to this issue involves the bedside label generation systems as described above for other laboratory specimens. These systems are compliant for pretransfusion sample collection, provided that the phlebotomist identification and specimen collection time are available to the blood bank when receiving the specimen.[103] This may require interfaces between the laboratory and blood bank computer systems when these systems are not provided by the same vendor.

Historically, crossmatching in the blood bank involved the use of serologic testing as a final check to ensure patient and donor red blood cell units are ABO compatible. An electronic method, the computer cross-match, has been demonstrated to be significantly more rapid and can provide additional safety when properly deployed.[104,105] In the computer cross-match, electronically stored, historical patient data are used to detect ABO incompatibilities between the ABO group of the patient's blood and the donor unit. There are stringent requirements for the safe use of the electronic cross-match that must be followed, including on-site validation of the system.[106]

Anatomic Pathology

Specimen Tracking

In anatomic pathology (AP), barcoding of the initially collected specimen can be a challenging proposition. Although AP orders may be ordered in CPOE systems, these orders are not generally transmitted to AP information systems, so laboratory-generated specimen labels are not available to be used for specimen labeling at the point of collection. In many cases, the specimen is labeled with a preprinted label containing only patient identifiers. Once the paper requisition and specimen information have been entered into the AP information system, the specimen container and requisition can be relabeled with barcodes containing the unique accession numbers for the case and the specimen. The safety of the subsequent workflow of the pathology laboratory may be enhanced by barcoding and scanning of specimen assets, including cassettes and slides.[64,107] Because of the limited space available on cassettes and slide labels, the barcodes used in AP in many cases may need to be 2D barcodes. Barcoded assets should be labeled in real time without the use of preprinted labels. Barcodes on cassettes and slides can facilitate the detailed tracking of these assets as they transit through pathology laboratories. In addition to preventing patient identification errors, asset tracking can assist with workflow analysis and identify process bottlenecks. RFID technology has shown promise in AP specimen tracking because the passive nature of the scanning and tracking possible with RFID tags has advantages over barcodes, which must be scanned at each step in the process.[108]

Summary

For many tests, the application of automation and rules-based approaches has made routine, within-laboratory testing processes more standardized and less error prone. However, significant patient safety gaps remain in all phases of laboratory testing, including ordering, collection, analysis, reporting, and interpretation. Technology can be increasingly incorporated into these processes to improve patient safety. It is important to note that the introduction of technology does not necessarily lead to improved or even unchanged patient safety because many technologies may have novel, often underappreciated failure modes. Improperly tested or implemented technologies can impair patient safety. Moreover, removal of the human element from a complex process can also remove the ability to identify an error. In this chapter, although technology to improve patient safety has been the primary focus, it is important to appreciate that technology can potentially introduce novel failure modes, and there is a need for monitoring, testing, and attention to downtime processes to ensure the selected technology has been implemented in a safe and durable manner.

References

1. Lippi G, Chance JJ, Church S, et al. Preanalytical quality improvement: from dream to reality. *Clin Chem Lab Med.* 2011;49(7):1113-1126.
2. Lippi G, Guidi GC, Mattiuzzi C, Plebani M. Preanalytical variability: the dark side of the moon in laboratory testing. *Clin Chem Lab Med.* 2006;44(4):358-365.
3. Plebani M. The detection and prevention of errors in laboratory medicine. *Ann Clin Biochem.* 2010;47(pt 2):101-110.
4. Laposata M, Dighe A. "Pre-pre" and "post-post" analytical error: high-incidence patient safety hazards involving the clinical laboratory. *Clin Chem Lab Med.* 2007;45(6):712-719.
5. Valenstein P, Meier F. Outpatient order accuracy. A College of American Pathologists Q-Probes study of requisition order entry accuracy in 660 institutions. *Arch Pathol Lab Med.* 1999;123(12):1145-1150.
6. Hickner J, Thompson PJ, Wilkinson T, et al. Primary care physicians' challenges in ordering clinical laboratory tests and interpreting results. *J Am Board Fam Med.* 2014;27(2):268-274.
7. Konrad TR, Link CL, Shackelton RJ, et al. It's about time: physicians' perceptions of time constraints in primary care medical practice in three national healthcare systems. *Med Care.* 2010;48(2):95-100.
8. Blumenthal D, Tavenner M. The "meaningful use" regulation for electronic health records. *N Engl J Med.* 2010;363(6):501-504.
9. Baron JM, Dighe AS. Computerized provider order entry in the clinical laboratory. *J Pathol Inform.* 2011;2:35.
10. Henricks WH, Wilkerson ML, Castellani WJ, Whitsitt MS, Sinard JH. Pathologists as stewards of laboratory information. *Arch Pathol Lab Med.* 2015;139(3):332-337.
11. Henricks WH, Wilkerson ML, Castellani WJ, Whitsitt MS, Sinard JH. Pathologists' place in the electronic health record landscape. *Arch Pathol Lab Med.* 2015;139(3):307-310.
12. Georgiou A, Westbrook JI. Computerised order entry systems and pathology services: a synthesis of the evidence. *Clin Biochem Rev.* 2006;27(2):79-87.
13. Thompson W, Dodek PM, Norena M, Dodek J. Computerized physician order entry of diagnostic tests in an intensive care unit is associated with improved timeliness of service. *Crit Care Med.* 2004;32(6):1306-1309.
14. Westbrook JI, Georgiou A, Lam M. Does computerised provider order entry reduce test turnaround times? A before-and-after study at four hospitals. *Stud Health Technol Inform.* 2009;150:527-531.

15. Grisson R, Kim JY, Brodsky V, et al. A novel class of laboratory middleware; promoting information flow and improving computerized provider order entry. *Am J Clin Pathol.* 2010;133(6):860-869.
16. Shah NR, Seger AC, Seger DL, et al. Improving acceptance of computerized prescribing alerts in ambulatory care. *J Am Med Inform Assoc.* 2006;13(1):5-11.
17. Kim JY, Dzik WH, Dighe AS, Lewandrowski KB. Utilization management in a large urban academic medical center: a 10-year experience. *Am J Clin Pathol.* 2011;135(1):108-118.
18. Tierney WM, McDonald CJ, Martin DK, Rogers MP. Computerized display of past test results: effect on outpatient testing. *Ann Intern Med.* 1987;107(4):569-574.
19. Bates DW, Kuperman GJ, Jha A, et al. Does the computerized display of charges affect inpatient ancillary test utilization? *Arch Intern Med.* 1997;157(21):2501-2508.
20. Tierney WM, Miller ME, McDonald CJ. The effect on test ordering of informing physicians of the charges for outpatient diagnostic tests. *N Engl J Med.* 1990;322(21):1499-1504.
21. Feldman LS, Shihab HM, Thiemann D, et al. Impact of providing fee data on laboratory test ordering: a controlled clinical trial. *JAMA Intern Med.* 2013;173(10):903-908.
22. Lo HG, Matheny ME, Seger DL, Bates DW, Gandhi TK. Impact of non-interruptive medication laboratory monitoring alerts in ambulatory care. *J Am Med Inform Assoc.* 2009;16(1):66-71.
23. Baron JM, Lewandrowski KB, Kamis IK, Singh B, Belkziz SM, Dighe AS. A novel strategy for evaluating the effects of an electronic test ordering alert message: optimizing cardiac marker use. *J Pathol Inform.* 2012;3:3.
24. Ash JS, Sittig DF, Campbell EM, Guappone KP, Dykstra RH. Some unintended consequences of clinical decision support systems. *AMIA Annu Symp Proc.* Oct 2007:26-30.
25. Kuperman GJ, Diamente R, Khatu V, et al. Managing the alert process at NewYork-Presbyterian Hospital. *AMIA Annu Symp Proc.* 2005:415-419.
26. Chan AJ, Chan J, Cafazzo JA, et al. Order sets in health care: a systematic review of their effects. *Int J Technol Assess Health Care.* 2012;28(3):235-240.
27. Rana R, Afessa B, Keegan MT, et al. Evidence-based red cell transfusion in the critically ill: quality improvement using computerized physician order entry. *Crit Care Med.* 2006;34(7):1892-1897.
28. Wang TJ, Mort EA, Nordberg P, et al. A utilization management intervention to reduce unnecessary testing in the coronary care unit. *Arch Intern Med.* 2002;162(16):1885-1890.
29. Chan J, Shojania KG, Easty AC, Etchells EE. Usability evaluation of order sets in a computerised provider order entry system. *BMJ Qual Saf.* 2011;20(11):932-940.
30. Leu MG, Morelli SA, Chung OY, Radford S. Systematic update of computerized physician order entry order sets to improve quality of care: a case study. *Pediatrics.* 2013;131(Suppl 1):S60-S67.
31. Overhage JM, Tierney WM, Zhou XH, McDonald CJ. A randomized trial of "corollary orders" to prevent errors of omission. *J Am Med Inform Assoc.* 1997;4(5):364-375.
32. Georgiou A, Williamson M, Westbrook JI, Ray S. The impact of computerised physician order entry systems on pathology services: a systematic review. *Int J Med Inform.* 2007;76(7):514-529.
33. Kuperman GJ, Gibson RF. Computer physician order entry: benefits, costs, and issues. *Ann Intern Med.* 2003;139(1):31-39.
34. Mutimer D, McCauley B, Nightingale P, Ryan M, Peters M, Neuberger J. Computerised protocols for laboratory investigation and their effect on use of medical time and resources. *J Clin Pathol.* 1992;45(7):572-574.
35. Nightingale PG, Peters M, Mutimer D, Neuberger JM. Effects of a computerised protocol management system on ordering of clinical tests. *Qual Health Care.* 1994;3(1):23-28.
36. Shalev V, Chodick G, Heymann AD. Format change of a laboratory test order form affects physician behavior. *Int J Med Inform.* 2009;78(10):639-644.
37. Peute LW, Aarts J, Bakker PJ, Jaspers MW. Anatomy of a failure: a sociotechnical evaluation of a laboratory physician order entry system implementation. *Int J Med Inform.* 2010;79(4):e58-e70.
38. Sinard JH, Castellani WJ, Wilkerson ML, Henricks WH. Stand-alone laboratory information systems versus laboratory modules incorporated in the electronic health record. *Arch Pathol Lab Med.* 2015;139(3):311-318.
39. Borycki EM. Technology-induced errors: where do they come from and what can we do about them? *Stud Health Technol Inform.* 2013;194:20-26.
40. Borycki EM, Kushniruk A, Keay E, Nicoll J, Anderson J, Anderson M. Toward an integrated simulation approach for predicting and preventing technology-induced errors in healthcare: implications for healthcare decision-makers. *Healthc Q.* 2009;12 Spec No Patient:90-96.
41. Garg AX, Adhikari NK, McDonald H, et al. Effects of computerized clinical decision support systems on practitioner performance and patient outcomes: a systematic review. *JAMA.* 2005;293(10):1223-1238.
42. Bates DW, Teich JM, Lee J, et al. The impact of computerized physician order entry on medication error prevention. *J Am Med Inform Assoc.* 1999;6(4):313-321.
43. Louis DN, Gerber GK, Baron JM, et al. Computational pathology: an emerging definition. *Arch Pathol Lab Med.* 2014;138(9):1133-1138.
44. Louis DN, Feldman M, Carter AB, et al. Computational pathology: a path ahead. *Arch Pathol Lab Med.* 2016;140:41-50.
45. Baron JM, Mermel CH, Lewandrowski KB, Dighe AS. Detection of preanalytic laboratory testing errors using a statistically guided protocol. *Am J Clin Pathol.* 2012;138(3):406-413.
46. Hill PM, Mareiniss D, Murphy P, et al. Significant reduction of laboratory specimen labeling errors by implementation of an electronic ordering system paired with a bar-code specimen labeling process. *Ann Emerg Med.* 2010;56(6):630-636.

47. Morrison AP, Tanasijevic MJ, Goonan EM, et al. Reduction in specimen labeling errors after implementation of a positive patient identification system in phlebotomy. *Am J Clin Pathol.* 2010;133(6):870-877.
48. Turner HE, Deans KA, Kite A, Croal BL. The effect of electronic ordering on pre-analytical errors in primary care. *Ann Clin Biochem.* 2013;50(Pt 5):485-488.
49. Hayden RT, Patterson DJ, Jay DW, et al. Computer-assisted bar-coding system significantly reduces clinical laboratory specimen identification errors in a pediatric oncology hospital. *J Pediatr.* 2008;152(2):219-224.
50. Bologna LJ, Mutter M. Life after phlebotomy deployment: reducing major patient and specimen identification errors. *J Healthc Inf Manag.* 2002;16(1):65-70.
51. Morrison AP, Melanson SE, Carty MG, Bates DW, Szumita PM, Tanasijevic MJ. What proportion of vancomycin trough levels are drawn too early?: frequency and impact on clinical actions. *Am J Clin Pathol.* 2012;137(3):472-478.
52. Melanson SE, Mijailovic AS, Wright AP, Szumita PM, Bates DW, Tanasijevic MJ. An intervention to improve the timing of vancomycin levels. *Am J Clin Pathol.* 2013;140(6):801-806.
53. Chen P, Tanasijevic MJ, Schoenenberger RA, Fiskio J, Kuperman GJ, Bates DW. A computer-based intervention for improving the appropriateness of antiepileptic drug level monitoring. *Am J Clin Pathol.* 2003;119(3):432-438.
54. Lippi G, Plebani M. Continuous-flow automation and hemolysis index: a crucial combination. *J Lab Autom.* 2013;18(2):184-188.
55. Lippi G, Ippolito L, Favaloro EJ. Technical evaluation of the novel preanalytical module on instrumentation laboratory ACL TOP: advancing automation in hemostasis testing. *J Lab Autom.* 2013;18(5):382-390.
56. Lima-Oliveira G, Lippi G, Salvagno GL, et al. Does laboratory automation for the preanalytical phase improve data quality? *J Lab Autom.* 2013;18(5):375-381.
57. Armbruster DA, Overcash DR, Reyes J. Clinical Chemistry Laboratory Automation in the 21st Century - Amat Victoria curam (Victory loves careful preparation). *Clin Biochem Rev.* 2014;35(3):143-153.
58. Holland LL, Smith LL, Blick KE. Total laboratory automation can help eliminate the laboratory as a factor in emergency department length of stay. *Am J Clin Pathol.* 2006;125(5):765-770.
59. Vermeer HJ, Thomassen E, de Jonge N. Automated processing of serum indices used for interference detection by the laboratory information system. *Clin Chem.* 2005;51(1):244-247.
60. Sepulveda JL, Young DS. The ideal laboratory information system. *Arch Pathol Lab Med.* 2013;137(8):1129-1140.
61. Jones JB. A strategic informatics approach to autoverification. *Clin Lab Med.* 2013;33(1):161-181.
62. Snyder SR, Favoretto AM, Derzon JH, et al. Effectiveness of barcoding for reducing patient specimen and laboratory testing identification errors: a laboratory medicine best practices systematic review and meta-analysis. *Clin Biochem.* 2012;45(13-14):988-998.
63. Hong MK, Yao HH, Pedersen JS, et al. Error rates in a clinical data repository: lessons from the transition to electronic data transfer: a descriptive study. *BMJ Open.* 2013;3(5):e002406.
64. Hanna MG, Pantanowitz L. Bar coding and tracking in pathology. *Surg Pathol Clin.* 2015;8(2):123-135.
65. Howanitz PJ. Errors in laboratory medicine: practical lessons to improve patient safety. *Arch Pathol Lab Med.* 2005;129(10):1252-1261.
66. Straseski JA, Strathmann FG. Patient data algorithms. *Clin Lab Med.* 2013;33(1):147-160.
67. Strathmann FG, Baird GS, Hoffman NG. Simulations of delta check rule performance to detect specimen mislabeling using historical laboratory data. *Clin Chim Acta.* 2011;412(21-22):1973-1977.
68. Baron JM, Cheng XS, Bazari H, et al. Enhanced creatinine and estimated glomerular filtration rate reporting to facilitate detection of acute kidney injury. *Am J Clin Pathol.* 2015;143(1):42-49.
69. Miller I. Development and evaluation of a logical delta check for identifying erroneous blood count results in a tertiary care hospital. *Arch Pathol Lab Med.* 2015;139(8):1042-1047.
70. Torke N, Boral L, Nguyen T, Perri A, Chakrin A. Process improvement and operational efficiency through test result autoverification. *Clin Chem.* 2005;51(12):2406-2408.
71. Fryer AA, Smellie WS. Managing demand for laboratory tests: a laboratory toolkit. *J Clin Pathol.* 2013;66(1):62-72.
72. Murff HJ, Gandhi TK, Karson AK, et al. Primary care physician attitudes concerning follow-up of abnormal test results and ambulatory decision support systems. *Int J Med Inform.* 2003;71(2-3):137-149.
73. Poon EG, Gandhi TK, Sequist TD, Murff HJ, Karson AS, Bates DW. "I wish I had seen this test result earlier!": dissatisfaction with test result management systems in primary care. *Arch Intern Med.* 2004;164(20):2223-2228.
74. Wilkerson ML, Henricks WH, Castellani WJ, Whitsitt MS, Sinard JH. Management of laboratory data and information exchange in the electronic health record. *Arch Pathol Lab Med.* 2015;139(3):319-327.
75. Lundberg G. When to panic over abnormal values. *MLO Med Lab Obs.* 1972;4:47–54.
76. Liebow EB, Derzon JH, Fontanesi J, et al. Effectiveness of automated notification and customer service call centers for timely and accurate reporting of critical values: a laboratory medicine best practices systematic review and meta-analysis. *Clin Biochem.* 2012;45(13-14):979-987.
77. Piva E, Pelloso M, Penello L, Plebani M. Laboratory critical values: automated notification supports effective clinical decision making. *Clin Biochem.* 2014;47(13-14):1163-1168.
78. Guidi GC, Poli G, Bassi A, Giobelli L, Benetollo PP, Lippi G. Development and implementation of an automatic system for verification, validation and delivery of laboratory test results. *Clin Chem Lab Med.* 2009;47(11):1355-1360.

79. Etchells E, Adhikari NK, Cheung C, et al. Real-time clinical alerting: effect of an automated paging system on response time to critical laboratory values: a randomised controlled trial. *Qual Saf Health Care*. 2010;19(2):99-102.
80. Lacson R, Prevedello LM, Andriole KP, et al. Four-year impact of an alert notification system on closed-loop communication of critical test results. *AJR Am J Roentgenol*. 2014;203(5):933-938.
81. Roy CL, Rothschild JM, Dighe AS, et al. An initiative to improve the management of clinically significant test results in a large health care network. *Jt Comm J Qual Patient Saf*. 2013;39(11):517-527.
82. Roy CL, Poon EG, Karson AS, et al. Patient safety concerns arising from test results that return after hospital discharge. *Ann Intern Med*. 2005;143(2):121-128.
83. Liao JM, Roy CL, Eibensteiner K, Nolido N, Schnipper JL, Dalal AK. Lost in transition: discrepancies in how physicians perceive the actionability of the results of tests pending at discharge. *J Hosp Med*. 2014;9(6):407-409.
84. Jones CD, Vu MB, O'Donnell CM, et al. A failure to communicate: a qualitative exploration of care coordination between hospitalists and primary care providers around patient hospitalizations. *J Gen Intern Med*. 2015;30(4):417-424.
85. El-Kareh R, Roy C, Brodsky G, Perencevich M, Poon EG. Incidence and predictors of microbiology results returning postdischarge and requiring follow-up. *J Hosp Med*. 2011;6(5):291-296.
86. Davenport TH, Glaser J. Just-in-time delivery comes to knowledge management. *Harvard Bus Rev*. 2002;80(7):107-111, 126.
87. Cimino JJ. Infobuttons: anticipatory passive decision support. *AMIA Annu Symp Proc*. 2008:1203-1204.
88. Del Fiol G, Cimino JJ, Maviglia SM, Strasberg HR, Jackson BR, Hulse NC. A large-scale knowledge management method based on the analysis of the use of online knowledge resources. *AMIA Annu Symp Proc*. 2010;2010:142-146.
89. Maviglia SM, Yoon CS, Bates DW, Kuperman G. KnowledgeLink: impact of context-sensitive information retrieval on clinicians' information needs. *J Am Med Inform Assoc*. 2006;13(1):67-73.
90. Challand GS, Vasikaran SD. The assessment of interpretation in clinical biochemistry: a personal view. *Ann Clin Biochem*. 2007;44(pt 2):101-105.
91. Lim EM, Sikaris KA, Gill J, et al. Quality assessment of interpretative commenting in clinical chemistry. *Clin Chem*. 2004;50(3):632-637.
92. Marshall WJ, Challand GS. Provision of interpretative comments on biochemical report forms. *Ann Clin Biochem*. 2000;37(Pt 6):758-763.
93. Vasikaran SD. Anatomy and history of an external quality assessment program for interpretative comments in clinical biochemistry. *Clin Biochem*. 2015;48(7-8):467-471.
94. Van Cott EM. Laboratory test interpretations and algorithms in utilization management. *Clin Chim Acta*. 2014;427:188-192.
95. Laposata ME, Laposata M, Van Cott EM, Buchner DS, Kashalo MS, Dighe AS. Physician survey of a laboratory medicine interpretive service and evaluation of the influence of interpretations on laboratory test ordering. *Arch Pathol Lab Med*. 2004;128(12):1424-1427.
96. Lewandrowski K, Gregory K, Macmillan D. Assuring quality in point-of-care testing: evolution of technologies, informatics, and program management. *Arch Pathol Lab Med*. 2011;135(11):1405-1414.
97. Nichols JH, Bartholomew C, Brunton M, et al. Reducing medical errors through barcoding at the point of care. *Clin Leadersh Manag Rev*. 2004;18(6):328-334.
98. Gilliss BM, Looney MR, Gropper MA. Reducing noninfectious risks of blood transfusion. *Anesthesiology*. 2011;115(3):635-649.
99. Nuttall GA, Stubbs JR, Oliver WC Jr. Transfusion errors: causes, incidence, and strategies for prevention. *Curr Opin Anaesthesiol*. 2014;27(6):657-659.
100. Novis DA, Miller KA, Howanitz PJ, Renner SW, Walsh MK. Audit of transfusion procedures in 660 hospitals: a College of American Pathologists Q-Probes study of patient identification and vital sign monitoring frequencies in 16494 transfusions. *Arch Pathol Lab Med*. 2003;127(5):541-548.
101. Bates DW, Cohen M, Leape LL, Overhage JM, Shabot MM, Sheridan T. Reducing the frequency of errors in medicine using information technology. *J Am Med Inform Assoc*. 2001;8(4):299-308.
102. Dzik WH. New technology for transfusion safety. *Br J Haematol*. 2007;136(2):181-190.
103. Dzik WH, Corwin H, Goodnough LT, et al. Patient safety and blood transfusion: new solutions. *Transfus Med Rev*. 2003;17(3):169-180.
104. Butch SH, Judd WJ, Steiner EA, Stoe M, Oberman HA. Electronic verification of donor-recipient compatibility: the computer crossmatch. *Transfusion*. 1994;34(2):105-109.
105. White MJ, Hazard SW III, Frank SM, et al. The evolution of perioperative transfusion testing and blood ordering. *Anesth Analg*. 2015;120(6):1196-1203.
106. Judd WJ. Requirements for the electronic crossmatch. *Vox Sang*. 1998;74(Suppl 2):409-417.
107. Pantanowitz L, Mackinnon AC Jr, Sinard JH. Tracking in anatomic pathology. *Arch Pathol Lab Med*. 2013;137(12):1798-1810.
108. Bostwick DG. Radiofrequency identification specimen tracking in anatomical pathology: pilot study of 1067 consecutive prostate biopsies. *Ann Diagn Pathol*. 2013;17(5):391-402.

6

Tools and Methods to Improve and Evaluate Patient Safety in the Laboratory

Tina Ipe, MD, MPH
Lee Hilborne, MD, MPH

Bringing Statistical Process Control From Industry to the Laboratory

As the Institute of Medicine challenged health care in 2000 to improve safety, the report and experts turned to safety lessons learned from other industries. The initial reaction of many when safety in health care was compared to safety in industries such as aviation and nuclear power was that health care is sufficiently different and more complex. Although this may be true, many of the processes and considerations employed by other industries are equally applicable to health care and specifically to laboratory medicine. For example, aviation regulations prevent airline pilots from performing "sunrise turnarounds" (ie, flying an additional leg after an overnight long-duration flight). The recognition that professionals who are tired are more error prone when lacking sleep is certainly not unique to aviation. The pathologist or laboratory professional who works a night shift should not be, except in extreme circumstances, expected to work the following day shift without sleep (the laboratory medicine equivalent to a sunrise turnaround).

Most laboratory professionals are familiar with using statistical processes to assure quality in the laboratory. Daily quality control procedures compare an analyte's performance to an established range that is based on expected values determined during the time of reagent validation (or verification). When the pathologist or laboratory supervisor reviews results from a recent College of American Pathologists (CAP) proficiency testing challenge, the laboratory's performance is compared to a statistically determined acceptable range that is based on the aggregate responses of all laboratories employing similar test systems responding to the same challenge.

Statistically, variation is commonly divided into *common cause variation* and *special cause variation*. Common cause variation is the normal or expected variation that is observed in any process. Well-controlled processes seek to reduce the common cause variation (ie, tighter standard deviation from the mean in a Gaussian distribution). Special cause variation is that which occurs outside the normal or expected process variation. This occurs when there are unexpected occurrences that are not predictable during normal operations.

There are a number of statistical approaches to evaluate errors and monitor laboratory quality. A few of them are discussed below.

Flow Charts. In response to an error or when analyzing a process, it is often invaluable to diagram the entire process. The act of diagramming the process and discussing it as a team serves several purposes.

- The diagram makes the process explicit. Frequently, when developing or discussing a flow diagram, different team members may disagree about the steps involved in the process. The diagram may reveal differences in interpretation or weaknesses in a standardized procedure that resulted in inconsistencies among facilities or personnel over time.
- The steps in the process that are explicit can then be evaluated with respect to the risk that they present for future failures or that contributed to an event being discussed (eg, failure mode and effects analysis or root cause analysis [RCA]). This allows for an objective assessment of each step in a process, facilitating identification of risk points that may have gone unrecognized. During a retrospective review of an adverse event, the recognition of an unsafe situation, even if not contributory to the immediate event, should be addressed. This is because the goal of any assessment, either prospective or retrospective, is to prevent the next adverse situation from occurring.
- A flow chart can be instrumental for reviewing a standard procedure with staff and for training new staff. Once there is agreement on the flow chart, the document may also be employed during period procedure review and competency assessment of staff.

Control Charting or Run Charting. Sometimes a "picture is worth a thousand words," and control charting is an approach that graphically displays how a process changes over time (Figure 6-1). Laboratorians are very familiar with control charts because it is common practice to display ongoing quality control data using a Levey-Jennings control chart. Although the plotting and interpretative processes have now been automated by some instruments, the resultant graphic display and the underlying data and interpretations are the same.

Tools and Methods to Improve and Evaluate Patient Safety in the Laboratory

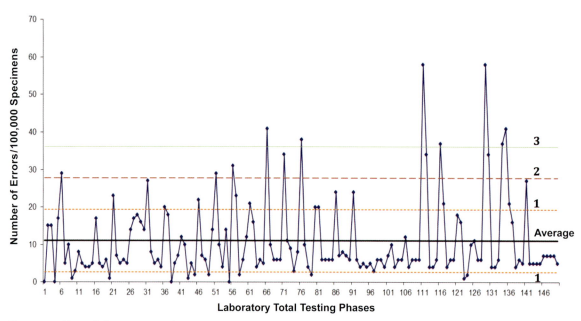

Figure 6-1. Control charting example.

The chart's y-axis is commonly centered around a mean value, and the ranges shown are defined in terms of 1, 2, and 3 standard deviations (SD). The x-axis represents time, with a result plotted for each control sample run. With each new result, the laboratory professional can compare that result to the findings already plotted on the chart and determine whether the process remains in control. This is commonly done by employing rules that "check" for common cause and special cause variation and look for unexpected trends in analytic performance.

Laboratories generally employ a set of statistical process rules by which to judge control performance. Variations on the Westgard set of rules can be found in most clinical laboratories.[1] We discuss here a few of the rules when using two levels of controls to illustrate how they may be applied in a manner to reduce common cause variation while quickly recognizing special cause variation so that corrective action can be taken.

1-3s rule (1 of 2 observations during a current run exceeds 3 SD). In most situations this represents a special cause variation, given that 99.7% of normal variation falls within 3 SD (ie, 3 in 1000 observations would be expected to yield a result greater than 3 SD from the mean by virtue of common variation). Laboratories often employ a 1-2s rule as a heads-up warning. No action on an initial violation of this rule would be taken because one would expect to observe this violation in 1 out of every 20 analyses performed (ie, 95% of observations would be expected to fall within 2 SD from the mean).

2-2s (both observations during a current run exceed 2 SD on the same side of the mean) and R-4s (both observations span more than 4 SD). Violations of these rules suggest that a process should be investigated for special cause variation. As before, this is an assessment based on probability. That is, the observations are sufficiently more likely to represent special cause variation than common cause variation. But that said, rarely does common cause variation produce these findings (eg, 2-2s would occur 0.25% by random chance alone).

It is also common to examine trends in control data over multiple observations. Frequent outliers that might, with one observation, be evaluated to be secondary to a one-time aberrant process must be questioned with more intense scrutiny when multiple observations show a similar repeat outlier. Similarly, observing 8 or 10 observations over time all on the same side of the mean suggests the possibility that the assay is drifting from the originally established mean.

Patient Safety Improvement Tools

The provision of safe, appropriate care to patients requires understanding the systems in which mistakes occur. Borrowing from successes in industries such as manufacturing, aeronautics, and nuclear power, health care has employed approaches and tools to reduce adverse medical events. For laboratory medicine, improvement of patient safety involves understanding the framework of the testing process, from specimen collection to producing an accurate test result. This framework is known as the *total testing process*[2] and includes the following steps:

1. Test selection and ordering of test
2. Patient identification
3. Specimen collection

4. Specimen transport to the clinical laboratory
5. Specimen preparation
6. Specimen analysis
7. Reporting test results
8. Test result interpretation
9. Action

Within this framework, patient safety tools in the clinical laboratory should be divided as tools for the collection of patient safety errors and tools for the analysis of patient safety errors.

Patient Safety Error Collection in the Laboratory

Errors occur in all phases of the total testing process. To determine the incidence of errors in all phases of the total testing process requires utilizing tools such as the following:

Event-Reporting Systems

This system relies on laboratory and health care personnel reporting events or issues that could impact patient safety.[3,4] This passive surveillance tool enables organizations to aggregate data on the incidence of errors and to gauge gaps in the workflow. The advantages are its relatively low cost and that workers who are involved and knowledgeable of the routine process are identifying safety issues. Negative aspects include a diversion of resources (employees) from other critical tasks and the propensity to place blame on an individual rather than on the system.

Surveillance Systems

Data collection of near misses and adverse events can also be performed through retrospective chart reviews, monitoring of high-risk workflow processes, and mining of electronic health records.[3] Insights garnered through these channels can lead not only to understanding the incident, but also help to prevent future patient-related safety concerns. Prospective patient safety tools involving data mining can also identify workflow system failures and prioritize efforts to prevent these failures.

Patient Safety Error Analysis

Lean Management

The origins of Lean management are in production/manufacturing, but it has recently been translated to the health care setting. The conceptualization of Lean is debatable: some argue it originated in the 1910s with the system implanted by Henry Ford called *flow production;* others believe it was conceptualized by Taiichi Ohno, who worked at Toyota's Honsha assembly plant in the 1940s. It was initially known as the *Toyota Production System (TPS).* Lean is considered an adaptation of TPS by many individuals, the principal goal of which is to eliminate non–value-added steps and processes. It is characterized by cycle time reduction, standardization, flexibility, and responding to customer needs. There are seven key areas of waste within manufacturing that are identified with this approach: overproduction, waiting, transport, motion, overprocessing, inventory, and defects. The Institute for Healthcare Improvement published a white paper on the application of Lean principles to health care,[5] in which it was noted that the core concept of Lean is to reduce waste and variation in systems. Health care is a complex and diverse setting because there is an interplay of many production processes, such as clinic visits, and players, including business entities and the patients themselves. Given the intricacy of health care, Lean has to be modified accordingly to this setting.[5]

Within the Lean management approach are key principles that are applicable to the clinical laboratory. These include tools such as: (1) value-added analysis and value stream mapping; (2) *kaizen*, which involves continuous process improvement with personnel engagement; (3) *kanban,* which serves as a guide for inventory management; and often (4) 5S (sort, set, shine, standardize, and sustain), which refers to physical redesign of the laboratory space to increase efficiency. In the laboratory, there are many processes that provide opportunities for improvement, such as quality control, proficiency testing, laboratory equipment, and customer satisfaction feedback. Lean management principles have been used to create a more efficient flow by adjusting the positioning of laboratory equipment. Streamlining the equipment process allows the laboratory to increase its testing capability and eliminate delays between steps.

Examples of the utility of Lean in the clinical laboratory were described by several clinical laboratories at Kaiser Permanante.[6] One such project was undertaken by the Department of Immunology and Virology at Kaiser Permanente and involved two different molecular assays. These assays involved testing in both departments and required laboratory personnel to travel between the two laboratories. Using a team-based approach, time-motion studies were conducted to determine metrics for productivity and staffing. Leadership was able to decrease personnel and equipment requirements, resulting in a successful implementation of coordinated testing. Another example was a study conducted by the Department of Bacteriology. The department had increased call volumes from physicians needing susceptibility results for blood culture isolates. The laboratory personnel reviewed the workflow pattern, reassigned this task to the blood culture bench, who then entered the culture results directly into the laboratory information system (LIS). Using

Lean methodology, workflow efficiency was increased, and incoming physician calls were decreased.

Along with the benefits of using the Lean approach in clinical laboratories, there are also some negatives. Challenges include the definition and collection of metrics to ensure sustainability of the approach; another is staff buy-in to the project.

Toyota Production System

As noted earlier, the Toyota Production System is the production/manufacturing system that was the basis of Lean management, in which (ideally) the output is defect free and is delivered in a timely manner to the customer. In addition, the work is done without waste in a safe and secure environment. An example of a health care organization using TPS is the Virginia Mason Medical Center in Seattle, Washington.[7] In 2001, the hospital was experiencing problems with patient safety and quality issues. They adopted TPS as their management system and conducted rapid improvement projects, kaizen, and 3P workshops. These changes resulted in increased patient quality of care, reduced hospital operating costs, decreased professional liability claims, and improved efficiencies in labor, space, and equipment.

Six Sigma

Six Sigma is another quality improvement approach that has been applied to health care. Similar to Lean management, it was initially created for the manufacturing industry by Motorola in 1979 and was adopted by health care organizations in the 1990s. The principal objective of this approach is to reduce errors using data and quantitative methods. This Greek term is used by statisticians to measure variation within a process, the ultimate goal of which is to have the measured process operating at 99.9996% perfection.[8] In particular, errors are to be decreased to 6σ level of 3.4 defects per million opportunities (DPMO). A process operating at a level of 6σ, producing 3.4 DPMO, is qualified as "world class." This approach uses the following five basic steps, with the acronym of DMAIC, to improve quality by decreasing the number of defects, reducing costs, and meeting customer expectations:

1. **D**efining the problem: Definition of the goals, customers, process owners, and stakeholders.
2. **M**easuring and collecting data: A quantitative measurement of the current system or process.
3. **A**nalyzing the sources for variation: Identification and elimination of gaps between current state and desired state.
4. **I**mproving the processes with variation: Changes implemented and evaluated quantitatively to determine if variation has been decreased.
5. **C**hecking for improvement by calculating the DPMO: Identification and formalization of newly implemented change into the operating procedures.

In the manufacturing industry, Six Sigma has reduced variation and improved processes, resulting in increased customer satisfaction and profitability; however, the same outcome has yet to be achieved in health care. Although it has been instituted in several global laboratories, in general laboratories have yet to achieve the Six Sigma goal for selected laboratory processes.[8] Although there is a dearth of published articles on the utility of Six Sigma in laboratory medicine, there have been documented drawbacks of this approach in the clinical laboratory.[9] Among them are the cost associated with implementing it in the laboratory, the need for highly trained technologists to lead these projects, selecting appropriate metrics, established cultural reticence, and issues of applying an industrial concept in a nonindustrial environment.[8,9]

In the few instances that laboratories used this approach and published their findings, errors were reduced, and cost savings and efficiency were increased. An example was the reduction of errors achieved by the North Shore–Long Island Health System Laboratory. This hospital's laboratory processes 3.5 million specimens annually.[10,11] Accessioning the laboratory specimens was an ongoing problem, with errors occurring in patient data entry, test ordering, and sample labeling. The goal of the project was to decrease data entry errors by 50% and to increase staff productivity. By using barcoded labels, the variance decreased, and patient safety and cost savings were increased.[10,11] Another example is the Froedtert Memorial Lutheran Hospital, where the Six Sigma approach was used to improve the turnaround time by 7.5 minutes and reduced laboratory loss of specimens by 35%.[10,12] These two examples illustrate that when projects within the laboratory are well defined, staff is involved and enthused about the project, and a project leader is identified who is familiar with the approach, laboratories can be successful in using Six Sigma to reduce process variations.

Plan, Do, Check, Act

This approach was created by Stewart and Deming, considered by many to be the founding fathers of quality control as a means to continually improve quality in business.[13] It was introduced to the health care field by the Institute for Healthcare Improvement. This methodology is a cyclical four-step model that is repeated again and again for continuous improvement. The rationale is that new changes fuel further process improvements. It is a tool that can be used when implementing a new quality improvement project, or new or improved design of process or service, or planning data collection and analysis.[14] The four phases, aligned with the DMAIC model discussed above, are as follows:

1. Plan: A process is identified for improvement. Strategies are developed to produce change.
2. Do: The proposed change is implemented.
3. Check (sometimes termed Study): The results of the change are analyzed. The results can be qualitative or quantitative.
4. Act: Take action and incorporate new insights. If the change(s) did not work, use a different solution to go through the cycle again.

Failure Mode and Effects Analysis

Failure mode and effects analysis (FMEA) is a prospective risk assessment tool that was developed by the military and the National Aeronautics and Space Administration.[15] It is used to determine potential failures or unrecognized hazards. The Department of Veterans Affairs and the National Center for Patient Safety introduced FMEA to health care organizations. The goal of this approach is to identify potential failures in processes and rectify them before the failures occur. Identification of failures employs flowcharts, Pareto diagrams, and fault trees.[16]

Flowcharts illustrate a process in sequential steps.[14] There are many types of flowcharts, including macro, top-down, detailed, and deployment flowcharts. Depending on the decision that needs to be made, each of these flowcharts has different applications and strengths.

A Pareto chart is a bar graph that is arranged with the longest bar on the left and the shortest bar on the right.[14] It helps to illustrate visually significant events, problems, or steps in a process. There are different types of Pareto charts, including nested, weighted, and comparative. A nested Pareto chart breaks a large category present in one graph into smaller subsections in a new second graph (Figure 6-2). A weighted Pareto chart is used to demonstrate relative importance of a

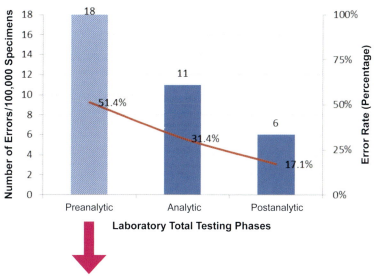
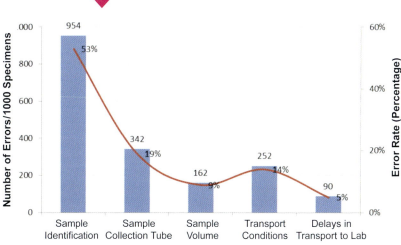

Figure 6-2. Example of a nested Pareto chart.

category. A comparative Pareto chart is used to compare two sets of data.

Fault tree analysis is used not only to identify root problems that lead to system failure, but also to identify changes that reduce risk of failure.[14] It is usually illustrated vertically with tree trunks at top and branches below.

An estimation determines the likelihood of the failure, the visibility of the failure, and the impact of the failure were it to occur. The estimate also helps to calculate and prioritize failures in terms of the likelihood and severity, also known as a risk priority number (RPN). Processes with low RPNs are error-free, whereas processes with high RPNs are generally complex with multiple steps.

An FMEA is conducted using the following steps[14]:
1. Select a project for FMEA analysis.
2. Assemble a multidisciplinary team with knowledge on the subject and the scope of the project, be it concept, system, design, process, or service.
3. Describe the project using flowcharts that detail functions, purpose, and end-user expectations.
4. For each process, identify potential failures and determine each failure severity (S) on a scale from 1 to 10 (1 = insignificant and 10 = catastrophic).
5. For each potential failure, determine the occurrence (O) rating, which is the probability of the failure to occur, also rated on a scale from 1 to 10.
6. For each potential failure, identify process controls that might prevent the cause from occurring and harming the patient. This detection rating (D) is also scored on a scale from 1 to 10.
7. Calculate the RPN = S × O × D. This ranks potential failures in the order they should be addressed.
8. Identify actions to reduce the risk of potential failures and thus the RPN.

FMEA was used by the Good Samaritan Hospital in 2001 to reduce risks associated with the process of blood product administration.[17] Reviewing the process flowchart helped to institute changes addressing the lack of access to blood products until a specific patient code was dialed. FMEA helped reduce and prevent patient safety errors related to blood product administration. The author did note that the process was time consuming, tedious, and difficult. Similarly, an FMEA project was conducted by six laboratories in South Korea as they transitioned from manual to automated blood grouping.[18] After a brief training session on FMEA, a comparison of manual versus automated blood grouping errors was performed. It showed that there was a decrease in RPN scores with the automated blood groupings when compared with manual groupings. Furthermore, the analysis identified steps within the automated process that had high RPNs that required additional review and redesign.

Root Cause Analysis

Root cause analysis (RCA) is a retrospective systematic review of an event with substandard outcomes. It was developed by the manufacturing industry to identify causal factors that produced industrial errors and later adapted by the health care industry to identify system deficiencies that led to medical errors. In sentinel events, many hospital associations and The Joint Commission ask that the health care organization submit an RCA with an action plan to rectify the root causes contributing to the error. The goal of the RCA is to determine the contributory factors of an event with the focus on the system rather than on individuals.

In laboratory medicine, Although RCAs are performed frequently, there is a dearth of documentation describing their utility. However, a qualitative analysis of 227 RCAs pertaining to the laboratory was performed at the Veterans Health Administration.[19] The analyses showed increases in RCAs from 1999 to 2008; two RCAs were performed in 1999 and 840 RCAs were completed in 2004. The study's authors reported that the analysis of the RCAs identified vulnerabilities in the total testing process of the Veterans Health Administration's laboratory medicine department. They also noted some benefits and challenges of using RCAs. The benefits are the narrative format of RCAs and the explanation of behavior that led to a particular negative outcome. The disadvantages of the RCA include limitations related to certain details, such as omission of important contributory clinical information. RCA usefulness is dependent on the team that provides the assessment and the person leading it, along with the limitation of hindsight bias. It is important to note that a thorough and credible RCA may identify other risk factors that were not directly contributory but nevertheless should be addressed by the organization to prevent future adverse events.

Another paper written by Diller et al[20] noted that patient safety gains have not occurred consistently with the use of RCAs in hospitals. According to these authors, RCAs are not effective because:
- There is no standardization in the RCA process between institutions. This makes interinstitutional comparisons difficult.
- A misguided focus is placed on the outcome and individual who caused the outcome rather than the systemic issues leading to that outcome.

- There is no implementation of an actionable corrective plan to correct the root causes.
- There is no collective summary of RCAs for the identification of trends. To be ideally used in health care, a standardized formatting and reporting of RCAs must occur. The RCA must explore the systemic issues that led to a poor outcome. RCAs must be collectively reviewed to identify trends.

Human Factors Analysis and Classification System

Based on Reason's theory that every organizational process is error prone and requires multiple barriers, Shappell and Wiegmann created the Human Factors Analysis and Classification System (HFACS).[20] It was used originally by the US Navy and Marine Corps but has since been adapted to other industries, including aviation, mining, and construction. It has also been used in health care settings to identify common root causes. The HFACS methodology for an adverse event is structured into the following four tiers, with subcategories for each[20]:

1. Unsafe act: An unsafe act is subcategorized as an error or violation. An error is defined as an accepted behavior that does not produce the desired outcome. In comparison, a violation is defined as a purposeful departure from accepted behavior.
2. Preconditions for unsafe acts: The operator's condition, personnel factors, and environmental factors are subcategories that help determine why the event occurred.
3. Supervision: This tier includes an understanding of the occurred error through subcategories such as leadership failure, operational planning, failure to correct existing problems, and ethics of supervisors.
4. Organizational influences: Errors can also result from the organization's structure, namely, the allocated resources, the climate of the organization, and the organization's processes.

Although HFACS has not been used in laboratory medicine, Diller et al[20] used the methodology at the Greenville Health System to prospectively review 105 adverse events. Based on their experience, the authors felt that when applied prospectively, this tool allowed for not only the identification of systemic and individual errors, but also the categorization of errors.

Laboratory Medicine–Based Patient Safety Tools

Because the aforementioned tools such as Lean management, FMEA, RCA, and others have been applied in isolation, they have failed to solve the problems of medical errors. Errors in the laboratory have been documented to occur in a range of 1 error per 164 results to 1 error per 8300 results.[21] Although errors do occur in laboratory medicine, when compared with other areas in medicine, laboratory medicine has a long history of focused efforts on improving quality. Because of regulations such as the Clinical Laboratory Improvement Amendments (CLIA) of 1988, clinical laboratories have worked hard to achieve goals such as specimen accuracy and reliability and timeliness of patient test results. Quality improvement projects began when concerned laboratorians noted that the quality of testing and its results were affected by processes that extended beyond the laboratory. Examples include processes such as test ordering, collection of the patient sample, and sample transportation to the laboratory.[22] Quality System Essentials (QSEs)—created by the American Association of Blood Banks (AABB) with adoption by the Clinical and Laboratory Standards Institute (CLSI)—are a quality tool that helps to analyze the technical activities of a laboratory. Performing quality control and proficiency testing helps to identify nonconforming events within the total testing process.

Quality System Essentials

QSEs were introduced by the AABB as a response to the Food and Drug Administration for mitigating the risks associated with bloodborne pathogens in blood products, namely, human immunodeficiency virus (HIV) in 1992.[23] It serves as a generic infrastructure management tool that supports the technical work performed by the laboratory. Given that the laboratory functions to transform a clinician's order into test results that can be used to diagnose and treat patients, the quality of the technical work is important in providing safe, effective, patient-centered, timely, efficient, and equitable patient care. There are 12 QSEs that are based on regulatory, accreditation, and standards requirements for the clinical laboratory. The 12 QSEs are as follows:
- Documents and records
- Organization
- Personnel
- Equipment
- Purchasing and inventory
- Process control
- Information management
- Occurrence management
- Internal and external assessments
- Process improvement
- Customer service and satisfaction
- Facilities and safety

Berte[23] modified the Quality Management System (QMS) model of the QSEs to reflect the regular updates by CLSI related to laboratory standards (Figure 6-3). She divided the QSEs into three groups to highlight the dynamic nature of the clinical laboratory: laboratory, work, and measurement. Regardless of the structure of the QSE framework, Berte proposes that tools such as Lean and Six Sigma be used in conjunction with the QSEs to sustain a culture of quality within the laboratory.

Q-Probes and Q-Tracks

The CAP created these tools starting in 1989 to improve the efficiency, efficacy, and quality of services provided by clinical pathology laboratories. Q-Probes is a voluntary survey composed of 10 features created by the Quality Practices Committee of the CAP.[24] After these surveys are developed, they are pilot tested in a few clinical laboratories before use by laboratories that want to participate in the survey. The Q-Probes survey allows participating laboratories to compare their performance to that of their peers. Interlaboratory performance is benchmarked as best, median, and most improvable performance for the participating laboratories. In comparison to the Q-Probes program, Q-Tracks allows for monitoring of laboratory quality over time rather than producing a single snapshot.[24,25] The following key indicators are monitored:

- Patient/specimen identification
- Stat test turnaround time
- Critical value reporting
- Specimen acceptability
- Customer satisfaction (general laboratory, anatomic laboratory)
- Corrected reports (general laboratory, anatomic laboratory)
- Surgical pathology/cytology specimen handling
- Blood product wastage
- Blood culture contamination

The goal of these quality indicators is clearly focused on learning from others to improve patient safety. When they are incorporated into a quality system that is already established in laboratory medicine, patient safety with regard to laboratory errors may improve.

Health Information Technology Tools

Patient safety can be affected by many errors, including overuse, underuse, and misuse of services. Another significant risk is the increased use of electronic health records (EHRs) in medical practices and institutions. Health information technology (HIT) expansion in medical practices and institutions was spurred by federal government regulations that will result in payment reduction penalties for the entities that do not incorporate EHRs. Given that computerized information systems have been utilized by both clinical and anatomic laboratories for decades, laboratory professionals can play vital roles in the selection of the EHR, especially with respect to the interface of the EHR to the laboratory information system (LIS). Key features of an LIS are that it interfaces well with the hospital's EHR and supports efficient laboratory operations while preserving patient safety and meeting regulatory requirements.[26]

The Institute of Medicine evaluated safety concerns with regard to HIT infrastructure in 2011. The committee found that the literature about HIT and patient safety was variable. However, EHR system safety was of overwhelming concern during a poll conducted by the Texas Medical Institute of Technology (TMIT). According to the Institute of Medicine, an effective HIT product has user-centered design principles that are tested and quality assured in actual or simulated clinical environments.[27] User-centered HIT has several salient features. It allows for the accurate and timely

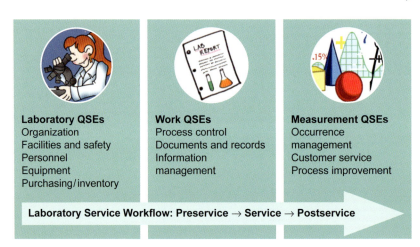

Figure 6-3. Quality System Essentials (QSEs). Modified from Berte.[23]

acquisition of data, thereby facilitating urgent decision making when needed. The data are formatted in a manner that is simple, easily understandable, and navigable. Other features include streamlining workflow, easy transfer of information, and no unanticipated downtime.

There are several tools to determine the safety of HIT, including simulators and self-assessments. An example of an EHR computerized patient order entry (CPOE) is the TMIT-EHR-CPOE flight simulator. This tool, according to Denham et al,[28] can verify performance of the HIT through simulation, has been used on a national scale to identify risks in HIT systems, and has helped health care organizations improve their HIT systems. It is important to test HIT systems because there might be glitches in the system that need to be addressed for the safety of the system and, ultimately, the patient. The TMIT-EHR-CPOE simulator tool performs evaluations remotely via a web-based format, quickly (within a matter of hours), and reliably. It uses seven steps, which are as follows[28]:

1. Registration for EHR-CPOE evaluation
2. Inputting test patient information
3. Inputting test orders
4. Entering orders into CPOE application
5. Submitting results
6. Scoring results
7. Reporting results

In addition to closing gaps in the HIT through simulation that might impact patient safety, assessments of the EHR-LIS interface are also important to evaluate patient safety because the LIS is only one component of the EHR system. Given the differences in functionalities of different EHRs, laboratory data transfer and integration may be jeopardized and may lead to poor patient safety outcomes. An important example is patient identification errors, which tend to occur in the preanalytic phase. These errors range from 1% to 2% for inpatients and from 0.2% to 6% for outpatients.[29] According to a CAP Q-Probes study, patient identification errors before verification of test results occurred 324 times per 1 million billable tests. Because many of these identification errors were caught before verification, there was a postverification frequency of 55 identification errors per 1 million billable tests.[29] To enable ease of selection and implementation of an LIS for the laboratory professional, an assessment tool called the LIS Functionality Assessment Toolkit is available. This toolkit provides the framework for reasoned decision making and includes functionalities such as software demonstration scenarios and the development of an ownership statement.[26] This assessment toolkit has four components[30]:

- An introductory report that guides toolkit use
- Approximately 850 weighted functionality statements
- Scripted scenarios to guide vendors during demonstrations
- Guidelines for determining the total cost of ownership

This tool will help medical directors choose an appropriate LIS system that satisfies the requirements of laboratory data as dictated in CLIA.

In addition to choosing the appropriate LIS system, it is paramount that the new or existing LIS interfaces well with the EHR system to minimize errors that affect patient safety. In efforts to optimize patient safety in the era of EHRs, the Office of the National Coordinator for Health Information Technology has released an assessment that helps health systems evaluate the safety of information systems within the EHR. This proactive assessment is called the *Safety Assurance Factors for EHR Resilience,* also known as the *SAFER Guides*. This assessment includes nine guidelines in the following areas[31]:

- High-priority practices
- Organizational responsibilities
- Contingency planning
- System configuration
- System interfaces
- Patient identification
- CPOE with decision support
- Test results reporting and follow-up
- Clinician communication

For each guideline, there is a checklist of recommended practices to determine the extent to which each recommendation has been instituted within the organization. The creators of the assessment recommend that a multidisciplinary team evaluate the potential HIT-related patient safety issues that might exist within their EHR system. As an example, if the test results reporting and follow-up guideline were implemented appropriately, diagnostic test results usage would be improved while mitigating undue risks to patients.

Summary

Patient safety initiatives require a multidisciplinary, systemic, transparent, blame-free approach. With the advent of proficiency testing in the 1940s, laboratory medicine has a longstanding dedication to quality patient care. Currently, laboratory medicine continues to play an integral role in keeping patients safe, with the utilization of many systems and tools, including Lean management, FMEA, QSEs, and Q-Probes, among others. Many of these tools were borrowed from other industries that have notable safety records and have been modified to fit health care needs. These tools not only help to identify problems, but to develop solutions to the problems. There have been many notable successes utilizing these tools in health care, including the use of Six Sigma at a hospital laboratory in New York and RCA at the Department of Veterans Affairs.

References

1. Westgard J, Westgard S. Designing SQC procedures. *Basic Quality Management Systems.* Madison, WI: Westgard QC; 2014.
2. Coskun A, Unsal I, Serteser M, Inal T. Six Sigma as a quality management tool: evaluation of performance in laboratory medicine. In: Coskun A, ed. *Quality Management and Six Sigma.* Rijeka, Croatia: InTech Publishers; 2010.
3. Wachter RM. Reporting systems, root cause analysis and other methods of understanding safety issues. In: Wachter RM, ed. *Understanding Patient Safety.* 2nd ed. New York, NY: McGraw-Hill; 2012. http://accessmedicine.mhmedical.com/content.aspx?bookid=396&sectionid=40414548. Accessed November 22, 2016.
4. Spell N. Tools to identify problems and reduce risk. In: McKean SC, Ross JJ, Dressler DD, Brotman DJ, Ginsberg JS. *Principles and Practice of Hospital Medicine.* New York, NY: McGraw-Hill; 2012. http://accessmedicine.mhmedical.com/content.aspx?sectionid=41303968&bookid=496. Accessed November 22, 2016.
5. Scoville R, Little K. *Comparing Lean and Quality Improvement.* Cambridge, MA: Institute for Healthcare Improvement; 2014.
6. Samuel L, Novak-Weekley S. The role of the clinical laboratory in the future of health care: lean microbiology. *J Clin Microbiol.* 2014;52:1812-1817.
7. Virginia Mason Production System. https://www.virginiamason.org. Accessed June 4, 2015.
8. Nevalainen D, Berte L, Kraft C, Leigh E, Picaso L, Morgan T. Evaluating laboratory performance on quality indicators with the six sigma scale. *Arch Pathol Lab Med.* 2000;124:516-519.
9. Landek D. Con: six sigma not always the right answer in the clinical laboratory. *Clin Leadersh Manag Rev.* 2006;20:E3.
10. Gras JM, Philippe M. Application of the Six Sigma concept in clinical laboratories: a review. *Clin Chem Lab Med.* 2007;45:789-796.
11. Riebling NB, Tria L. Laboratory toolbox for process improvement: Six Sigma at North Shore–Long Island Jewish Health System. *Lab Med.* 2008;39:7-14.
12. Simmons JC. Using Six Sigma to make a difference in health care quality. *Qual Lett Healthc Lead.* 2002;14:2-10, 1.
13. Moen R, Norman C. Evolution of the PDCA Cycle. http://pkpinc.com/files/NA01MoenNormanFullpaper.pdf. Accessed November 22, 2016.
14. Tague N. *The Quality Toolbox.* 2nd ed. Milwaukee, WI: American Society for Quality, Quality Press; 2005.
15. Chiozza ML, Ponzetti C. FMEA: a model for reducing medical errors. *Clin Chim Acta.* 2009;404:75-78.
16. Krouwer JS. An improved failure mode effects analysis for hospitals. *Arch Pathol Lab Med.* 2004;128:663-667.
17. Burgmeier J. Failure mode and effect analysis: an application in reducing risk in blood transfusion. *Jt Comm J Qual Improv.* 2002;28:331-339.
18. Han TH, Kim MJ, Kim S, et al. The role of failure modes and effects analysis in showing the benefits of automation in the blood bank. *Transfusion.* 2013;53:1077-1082.
19. Dunn EJ, Moga PJ. Patient misidentification in laboratory medicine: a qualitative analysis of 227 root cause analysis reports in the Veterans Health Administration. *Arch Pathol Lab Med.* 2010;134:244-255.
20. Diller T, Helmrich G, Dunning S, Cox S, Buchanan A, Shappell S. The Human Factors Analysis Classification System (HFACS) applied to health care. *Am J Med Qual.* 2014;29:181-190.
21. Stankovic AK. The laboratory is a key partner in assuring patient safety. *Clin Lab Med.* 2004;24:1023-1035.
22. Howanitz PJ, Perrotta PL, Bashleben CP, et al. Twenty-five years of accomplishments of the College of American Pathologists Q-Probes program for clinical pathology. *Arch Pathol Lab Med.* 2014;138:1141-1149.
23. Berte LM. Laboratory quality management: a roadmap. *Clin Lab Med.* 2007;27:771-790, vi.
24. Wagar EA, Tamashiro L, Yasin B, Hilborne L, Bruckner DA. Patient safety in the clinical laboratory: a longitudinal analysis of specimen identification errors. *Arch Pathol Lab Med.* 2006;130:1662-1668.
25. Howanitz PJ. Errors in laboratory medicine: practical lessons to improve patient safety. *Arch Pathol Lab Med.* 2005;129:1252-1261.
26. Henricks WH, Wilkerson ML, Castellani WJ, Whitsitt MS, Sinard JH. Pathologists' place in the electronic health record landscape. *Arch Pathol Lab Med.* 2015;139:307-310.
27. Committee on Patient Safety and Health Information Technology; Institute of Medicine. *Health IT and Patient Safety: Building Safer Systems for Better Care.* Washington, DC: National Academies Press; 2011.
28. Denham CR, Classen DC, Swenson SJ, Henderson MJ, Zeltner T, Bates DW. Safe use of electronic health records and health information technology systems: trust but verify. *J Patient Saf.* 2013;9:177-189.
29. Wilkerson ML, Henricks WH, Castellani WJ, Whitsitt MS, Sinard JH. Management of laboratory data and information exchange in the electronic health record. *Arch Pathol Lab Med.* 2015;139:319-327.
30. Sinard JH, Castellani WJ, Wilkerson ML, Henricks WH. Stand-alone laboratory information systems versus laboratory modules incorporated in the electronic health record. *Arch Pathol Lab Med.* 2015;139:311-318.
31. The Office of the National Coordinator for Health Information Technology. *SAFER Guides: Safety Assurance Factors for EHR Resilience.* January 2014. https://www.healthit.gov/safer/safer-guides. Accessed November 22, 2016.

7

Diagnostic Errors and Cognitive Bias

Stephen S. Raab, MD

Introduction

The cognitive activities of pathologists play a central role in the fields of anatomic and clinical pathology. Consequently, failures in cognition may result in errors that are associated with patient harm. This chapter examines cognitive activities in the broader perspective of work processes and uses quality management principles to deconstruct and understand the remarkable strengths (described as *Safety II*) and limitations (described as *Safety I*) of cognitive processes of pathologists in producing an accurate and precise diagnostic interpretation. This deconstruction provides the data on how pathologists assure safer practices and how redesign of systems could mitigate cognitive limitations.

Understanding Work

In the late 19th and early 20th centuries, the development of scientific management methods led to a greater understanding of work, with a goal of improving efficiency. Scientific management focused on redesigning the components of work process and spawned the growth of work-based quality management systems that involved the development of quality improvement and quality assurance structures.[1] Systems such as Fordism, Lean, and Total Quality Management are examples of management systems that arose from the early scientific management methods.[2-4]

The processes of work have been described in a number of ways. For example, Spear and Bowen[5] described the work *rules* (ie, component processes) of the Lean Toyota Production System as activities, connections (handoffs), and pathways (flow). A goal of management is to perform these work processes with a high level of quality. The Institute of Medicine (IOM) classified six domains of health care quality—safety, efficiency, effectiveness, equity, patient-centeredness, and timeliness of care—with a major emphasis being placed on patient safety.[6] Metrics have been established for each of these quality domains for many health care work processes. Medical error is a commonly used metric for patient safety.

By understanding the current state of work component processes, individuals trained in quality improvement and change methods are able to facilitate front-line personnel in optimizing the quality of all these processes.[7] Quality assurance activities develop a structure to maintain levels of high quality.

The work of pathologists occurs in a sociotechnological environment, in which work activities are performed by individuals and/or technologies. For individuals, work activities may be classified as technical (motor) and cognitive (brain). Cognition is the set of all mental abilities and processes related to knowledge, attention, memory, judgment, evaluation, problem solving, decision making, comprehension, and production of language.[8] In work, cognitive processes use existing knowledge and may generate new knowledge. Cognitive abilities are brain-based skills we use to complete almost any task. Table 7-1 lists examples of cognitive abilities and skills.[9]

All individuals practicing in anatomic or clinical pathology—including technologists, pathologist extenders, and support staff—perform both technical and cognitive work tasks on a daily basis. In order to examine the relationship of cognition and error, this chapter specifically focuses on pathologist diagnostic error in the field of anatomic pathology. This focus allows for a more detailed discussion of cognitive activities, including the cognitive processing of sensory stimuli in order to make a diagnosis.

Safety Science

The IOM defined a medical error to be a failure of a planned action to be completed as intended or the use of a wrong plan to achieve an aim.[10]

The concept of medical error is not new, as the Greeks long ago described iatrogenesis as the inadvertent and preventable induction of disease or complication by the medical treatment of a physician. The 2000 IOM report, *To Err is Human: Building a Safer Health System*,[10] highlighted that the current level of error was unacceptably high.

The IOM report spawned the patient safety movement and the investigation of the types, causes, frequency, classification, and consequences of medical error. From a work perspective, medical errors generally may be viewed as system process failures that occur in activities, handoffs, and patient flow.

In the field of patient safety, investigators have studied work processes from two perspectives. Safety I is the study of work from the perspective of what goes

Diagnostic Errors and Cognitive Bias

Table 7-1. Cognitive Abilities and Associated Skills	
Ability	**Skills**
Perception	Processing of sensory stimuli
Attention	Maintaining concentration on an action or thought and managing competing sensory demands
Memory	Utilizing short-term working memory and long-term memory
Motor skills	Mobilizing the body to manipulate objects
Language	Translating sounds into words
Spatial and visual processing	Specific processing of visual stimuli to understand relationship among objects
Higher-order functions	Skills that enable goal-oriented behavior, such as the ability to plan. These skills include the following: **Anticipation:** Prediction based on pattern recognition **Flexibility:** Capacity to switch mental modes **Problem solving:** Capacity to define a problem and potential solutions **Decision making:** Capacity to make decisions based on problem solving **Working memory:** Capacity to hold and manipulate information **Sequencing:** Capacity to break down complex actions into units and prioritize these units in the appropriate order **Inhibition:** Capacity to avoid distraction and internal urges

wrong (to cause the error) and is the classic frame described in the IOM report. Much of the anatomic pathology literature describes error from this perspective. Safety II is the study of what goes right and is the opposite of Safety I.[11] Many safety improvement initiatives originate from the understanding of systems that have work processes with fewer errors. For most health care work processes, things go wrong less than 5% of the time, but there has been little explicit study of the 95% of processes that go right. Safety II involves the study of system resilience, which has two definitions: (1) the ability to recover or adjust from change, misfortune, or adversity; and (2) the ability to return to the original form after been bent or stressed (elasticity).

From the scientific standpoint, an error is the difference between a set point (ie, the set point is where a process value should match) and a process value. Anatomic and clinical pathology laboratories have classified interpretive (diagnostic) errors as those of diagnostic accuracy (eg, failure to diagnose correctly or classify a disease process) and those of diagnostic precision (eg, failures in agreement on the diagnosis).[12] Anatomic pathology diagnostic errors most commonly are detected by some form of secondary review, where disagreements represent both imprecision and inaccuracy (at least for one of the diagnoses). Both Safety I and II stress the importance of examining error from the system perspective, which involves analytic, preanalytic, and postanalytic processes.

Much of the pathology Safety I literature has helped to define the current state of frequency of diagnostic error, based on different error detection methods. A commonly used method in this approach is secondary review practice, in which a second pathologist reviews the diagnostic interpretation of a first pathologist. This method is used in both anatomic and clinical pathology. This detection method generally is used to assess accuracy, although it also assesses precision. In anatomic pathology, Nakhleh et al[13] reported that the median discrepancy frequency based on secondary review practices (n = 137 published reports) was 18.3%, with a major median discrepancy frequency of 5.9%. In this study, the term *major* had several meanings, including demonstrated impact on care, potential impact on care, and substantial diagnostic differences. Solely on the basis of second institutional review (n = 41), Raab and Grzybicki[14] reported an overall case discrepancy frequency of 11.4%, with a major discrepancy frequency of 4.7%. Although these data are associated with case selection bias, two pathologists disagree with each other between 1 in 10 and 1 in 5 cases, with a major difference of opinion (potentially a sentinel or harmful event) in approximately 1 in 20 cases.

To better assess precision, investigators have reported interobserver variability frequencies in most organ systems, and kappa values range considerably and depend on specimen type, diagnostic cutoffs, level of expertise, and a number of other factors. For example, Wechsler et al[15] reported that the kappa statistic (95% confidence interval) for experts in the diagnosis of malignant melanoma in childhood ranged from 0.31 to 0.38. Kappa values may be higher than 0.80 for some diagnoses (tubular adenomas) but may be even lower than 0.20 for others. Raab et al[16] showed that pathologists exhibited poor agreement in the traditional assessment of error root cause (sampling versus interpretation), and the pairwise kappa statistic ranged from -0.154 to 1.

Pathology Work Process and Cognitive Failures

Pathology testing phases largely consist of technical-cognitive processes (ie, human activities involving technologies). For example, anatomic pathology personnel who perform gross tissue examination use a variety of technologies (eg, gross room benches, cutting instruments, electronic information systems) in their work. Pathologists also utilize a variety of technologies in order to render a diagnostic opinion on individual specimens.

Failures may occur at any process step and may involve a problem with the technology alone, cognition alone, or the cognitive-technical interaction. In 1990, Reason[17] categorized cognitive errors as either mistakes or slips. *Mistakes* are errors in choosing an objective or in specifying a method of achieving an objective. *Slips* are errors in carrying out an intended method for achieving the objective.[18] Norman[19] considered that the difference between a mistake and a slip was one of intention to act: a mistake occurs if the intention is not appropriate, whereas a slip occurs if the action is not what was intended.

An example of a gross tissue examination mistake is choosing the incorrect protocol for a specific specimen, such as using a benign colon block submission protocol for a colonic specimen with cancer. This is an example of choosing the wrong method to achieve an aim. An example of a gross examination slip is choosing the correct protocol but not submitting the correct number of tissue sections as required by the protocol. In this case, the correct method was chosen, but an error was made in carrying out the method.

Investigators have further subclassified slips. Sternberg[18] reported that slips may occur (1) when an individual is required to deviate from routine and intentional controlled processes are overridden by inappropriate automatic processes or (2) when automatic processes are interrupted either by external events or internal events (eg, distracting thoughts). This assessment involves assigning cause to classify slip type (ie, deviation versus interruption). Many medical slips fall in the second category and are a result of busy, hectic external and internal environments.

Traditionally, causal error classification systems have been developed to serve as a framework around which new investigative methods may be designed and existing accident error databases restructured. An example of this system is the Human Factors Analysis and Classification System (HFACS), developed largely by and for the aviation industry because human error has been implicated in 70% to 80% of all aviation accidents.[20] HFACS incorporates Reason's concepts of latent factors (ie, predisposing conditions that may lead to a failure) and the active failure itself. For example, a diagnostic or active failure in anatomic pathology (eg, interpreting a sample as benign when the sample actually shows malignancy) potentially may be associated with a number of preconditions or latent factors, such as hectic work environment, tiredness, or interruptions, which contribute to or are associated with the error.

HFACS describes active failures (Unsafe Acts) and three levels of latent factors (Preconditions for Unsafe Acts, Unsafe Supervision, and Organizational Influences). Unsafe Acts are subdivided into errors and violations. *Errors* are the mental or physical activities of personnel that fail to achieve an intended outcome. HFACS further categorizes errors as decision errors (mistakes), skill-based errors (slips), and perceptual errors (response failure to degraded or unusual sensory input). Examples of these errors and latent factors in pathology will be discussed below.

Violations are the willful disregard for the rules and regulations of practice and are further classified as *routine* (often referred to as bending the rules and implicitly accepted by management) and *exceptional* (extreme in nature and not condoned by management). For example, in anatomic pathology, a routine violation is a pathologist choosing not to perform a microscopic examination of a second tissue level when the first and third levels have the same histologic findings. An exceptional violation is a pathologist not completing a validation procedure when bringing on a new interpretive test and then signing off that the validation was completed. Shappell and Wiegmann[20] describe a routine violation in aviation as being similar to driving a car 64 miles per hour in a speed zone of 55 miles per hour and an exceptional violation as driving 105 miles per hour in a 55 miles per hour speed zone.

Other categorical error classification systems have been developed in non–health care domains and then applied to health care or have been developed in health care fields. These include the modified Eindhoven classification model (used in transfusion medicine and cytopathology)[21,22] and The Joint Commission (formerly Joint Commission on Accreditation of Healthcare Organization [JCAHO]) Patient Safety Event Taxonomy.[23] The JCAHO taxonomy includes five complementary root nodes or primary classifications: impact, type, domain, cause, and prevention and mitigation (Figure 7-1). Examples of anatomic and clinical pathology cognitive errors are shown in Table 7-2.

Pattern Recognition

On one level, pathologists are problem solvers and ascribe an interpretive categorization to bodily specimens that manifest a disease (or normal/nondisease)

Diagnostic Errors and Cognitive Bias

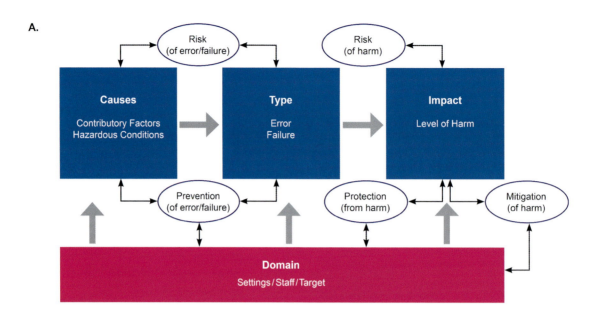

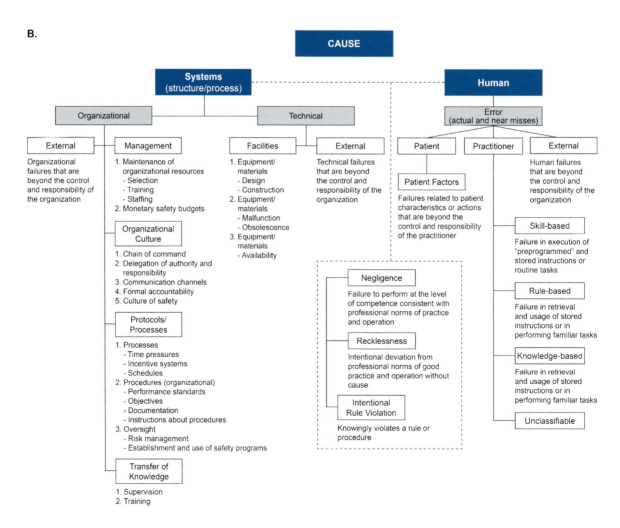

Figure 7-1. A. Joint Commission Patient Safety Event Taxonimy. B. Joint Commission classification of causes of error.

Table 7-2. Examples of Cognitive Errors in Anatomic and Clinical Pathology		
Classification Type	Anatomic Pathology	Clinical Pathology
Skill-based	Failure to examine entire frozen section slide, resulting in missing a small focus of tumor	In transfusion medicine, failure to confirm at bedside that the patient is getting the correct blood product
Rule-based	Failure to fully complete the College of American Pathologists' cancer checklist for a lung cancer specimen, resulting in a failure to report lymph node metastases	In chemistry, failure to adhere to the Westgard rules in quality control
Knowledge-based	In fine-needle aspiration of a thyroid gland, misinterpretation of a hyalinizing trabecular neoplasm as a papillary carcinoma	In microbiology, misinterpretation of a rarely seen organism

process. This categorization is based on cognitive decision-making processes. As in technical work, the cognitive decision-making process may be further examined in terms of internal mental activities, pathways, and connections, as well as external activities, pathways, and connections that affect the internal processes. Failures in these mental work processes may lead to errors.

A large body of literature has been published on human cognitive decision making, which is a complex process that involves many layers. This chapter primarily will examine the cognitive task of pattern recognition, which matches information from a stimulus to information retrieved from memory.

Investigators have proposed different theories of pattern recognition[24-26]:

- Feature analysis: Each stimulus (eg, sensory information) has a set of distinctive features or characteristics. The human sensory system breaks down incoming stimuli into these characteristics and then processes this information. One method of processing is assessing the characteristics that may be more important than others for recognition. This work process has the following four steps:
  1. Stimulus detection
  2. Pattern dissection into characteristics
  3. Comparison of stimulus characteristics to those in memory
  4. Recognition
- Template matching: A new stimulus is compared directly to copies (or templates) in long-term memory. Templates are stored in memory as part of the learning process. Recognition occurs when the new stimulus matches the template.[27]
- Prototype matching: A new stimulus is compared to a prototype, or a standard model of that stimulus. Unlike template matching and feature analysis, an exact match is not necessary, and recognition occurs when a similar prototype is found in memory.
- Recognition by components[28]: Individuals recognize objects by identifying main component parts (ie, geons), which are based on basic three-dimensional shapes (eg, cone, sphere). Geons are compared to objects in stored memory. This theory proposes that we focus on edges and the area where two edges meet (ie, concavities).

These theories describe the cognitive work of pattern recognition in different frames, and each theory has strengths and weaknesses when applied to pathologist pattern recognition. The building of *mental maps* of the knowledge of features, templates, and prototypes generally is a long-standing (even lifelong) activity, and the processes include optimally performing stepwise activities as mentioned above in the theory of feature analysis. If these stepwise cognitive activities are flawed, the use of the mental map also could lead to error.

Pathologist Cognition

Most medical practitioners use a form of pattern recognition when rendering a diagnostic opinion. Anatomic pathologists make interpretations of gross tissue and cellular level disease using the cognitive method of *image-based pattern recognition*. Clinical pathologists also use image-based pattern recognition in fields such as microbiology, flow cytometric analysis, and transfusion medicine. For a more detailed discussion, anatomic pathology pattern recognition will be discussed.

For this process at a cellular level, a pathologist makes a diagnosis of a specific disease by (1) visually examining a cellular-level image obtained from a patient's bodily tissue (stimulus detection), (2) breaking down the stimulus into component characteristics (eg, assessing for the presence of criteria), and (3) associating a specific combination of observed morphologic criteria with that specific disease (feature comparison and recognition). A pathologist may use additional data—such as clinical history, radiologic impressions, or other inputs—in the decision-making process. These data often construct a specific context in which the pattern recognition occurs.

Gross tissue examination also involves pattern recognition, which generally results in producing descriptive data that are used later in cellular disease decision making and inform sectioning protocols.

Pathologists generally learn gross and cellular-level pattern recognition in an apprenticeship environment in which pathologists with more expertise (masters) teach these patterns of criteria and the associated diagnosis of a specific disease to less experienced pathologists or trainees (novices).

Using the process of pattern recognition, a pathologist examines a tissue slide and looks for criteria of normality and abnormality within the tissue. Pattern recognition depends on linking the observed patterns of criteria with knowledge of mental maps of patterns of criteria that represent specific diseases. The presence of normal tissue in the same sample, for comparison, is often useful.

A criterion describes (1) a specific characteristic of a cell (eg, morphologic feature of color, size, shape); (2) the specific arrangement of cells (eg, small clusters, sheets, glandular-like structures); or (3) the specific tissue architecture or relationship of cellular and noncellular components (eg, invasion, necrosis, microcalcification). Table 7-3 shows examples of typical criteria observed in a patient who has cervical intraepithelial neoplasia 1 (CIN I). This is not an exhaustive list of criteria because, in actuality, the individual cells, cellular arrangements, and cellular relationships display a large variety of appearances.

Some criteria are more important than other criteria in making a diagnosis, as these criteria are more *representative* of a group of diseases or a specific disease.

A criterion may have a variable appearance within an individual case of a disease. Some of this variability is real and some is *artifact*, defined as an artificial product or effect introduced by technology used in a scientific investigation, such as a diagnostic or screening test. An example of an analytic process artifact is truncated nuclear structures secondary to tissue sectioning. Artifacts are introduced in both the preanalytic and analytic testing phases, and the recognition of the effect of artifact in pattern recognition is extremely important. The preanalytic steps of sampling (which alters size, shape, and gross and cellular features), tissue fixation, and processing are major factors that alter important criteria for all disease and nondisease states.

Variability in criteria is readily apparent in Figure 7-2, A, regarding the size of a CIN I cell nucleus, with some cell nuclei being large and other cell nuclei appearing smaller. A qualitative frequency distribution of CIN I nuclear size is shown in Figure 7-2, B. Investigators have further quantified the distribution of an individual criterion (eg, cell size, nuclear chromatin appearance, or mitotic frequency) for a variety of diseases.

Of course, criteria do not have the same frequency distribution among specimens from the population of patients who have the same disease. For example,

Table 7-3. Typical Criteria in Cervical Intraepithelial Neoplasia 1 (CIN I)	
Cellular Criterion	**Typical Appearance**
Nuclear component	
Size	• Large
Density of chromatin	• Hyperchromatic
Appearance of membrane	• Irregular
Distribution of chromatin	• Irregular
Cytoplasmic component	
Amount	• Moderate
Density	• High
Presence of vacuoles	• No
Color	• Red (keratinized)
Cell bridges	• Yes
Perinuclear clearing	• Irregular in contour
Cellular Arrangement Criterion	
Cell location	Base of epithelium
Cell height	Up to lower one-third of cell thickness
Tissue Architecture or the Relationship of Cellular and Noncellular Components Criterion	
Invasion	Absent
Basement membrane	Present
Stromal desmoplasia	Absent

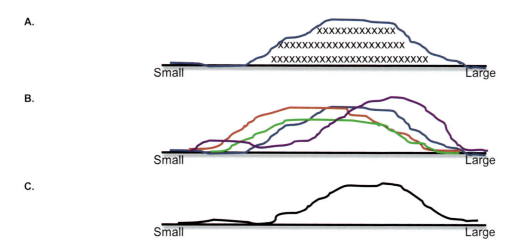

Figure 7-2. A. Qualitative representation of nuclear size in the cells of a cervical intraepithelial neoplasia 1 (CIN I). Each X represents the size of one cell nucleus. The curve represents the frequency distribution of nuclear size in all the cells in the specimen. B. Frequency distribution of nuclear size in four specimens of CIN I. C. Normalized frequency distribution of nuclear size in four specimens of CIN I.

Figure 7-2, C, shows the frequency distribution of nuclear size in specimens from four different patients who have CIN I. On the average, slides from some biopsy specimens of CIN I have more nuclei of larger size than other specimens—a single, fixed prototype (of the criterion of nuclear size) does not exist. For a malignancy such as an invasive cervical squamous cell carcinoma, the variation in nuclear size enters into the assessment of tumor differentiation (ie, well, moderately, or poorly differentiated).

Some diseases are considered to have well-defined histologic or cytopathologic variants, exemplifying the predominance of specific criteria. Other diseases have several well-known variants that display different prominent criteria. For example, histologic preparation of cervical biopsy tissue from a patient who has CIN I may show cells having convoluted nuclei that are typical of changes caused by human papillomavirus or nuclei showing the features of classic mild dysplasia. A cervical biopsy sample from a patient who has an invasive cervical squamous cell carcinoma may have a keratinized, nonkeratinized, or spindled cell appearance.

The combination of criteria is the pattern of the disease. An example of a qualitative disease pattern-of-criteria plot or *disease-pattern/spectrum* is shown in Figure 7-3, A, for the diagnosis of the *classic presentation* of low-grade squamous intraepithelial lesion (LSIL) on a liquid-based Papanicolaou (Pap) test. The *LSIL pattern/spectrum* generally is a template that is based on an expert's opinion or mental map, which, in turn, is based on that expert's apprenticeship training, experiences, and the large number of cases that the expert has examined in their practice. These templates generally are not firmly fixed and represent estimations of general patterns that are difficult to quantify.

Nonclassic presentations of a specific disease are caused by several factors, including patient-related factors (eg, unusual or rare disease morphologic presentation) and artifacts. The disease pattern spectrum of a population of nonclassic presentations of a specific disease may overlap with the spectrum of the classic presentation or represent an entirely different mental map.

In the current method of apprenticeship training, novices implicitly learn disease pattern spectra of a local expert mentor and from textbooks written by other experts. As the novice examines more and more patient specimens of classic and nonclassic presentations of disease, the novice *develops* their own disease pattern spectrum as a result of the process of learning, and it changes over time (and changes more dramatically for novices). The formation of disease pattern spectra stabilize as more patient specimens are encountered.

Figure 7-3, B, shows an expert's two disease pattern spectra of within-normal-limits (WNL) Pap tests and of LSIL Pap tests. The green line is the expert's threshold of separation of normal from LSIL based on the pattern of criteria. In reality, this threshold is not firm but may change subtly on a frequent basis. This borderline may further be altered by inclusion of diagnoses of greater uncertainty (eg, atypical cells of undetermined significance or neither WNL or LSIL).

Diagnostic Errors and Cognitive Bias

A.

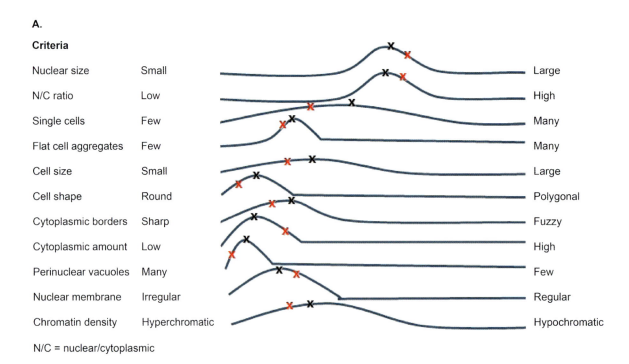

B.

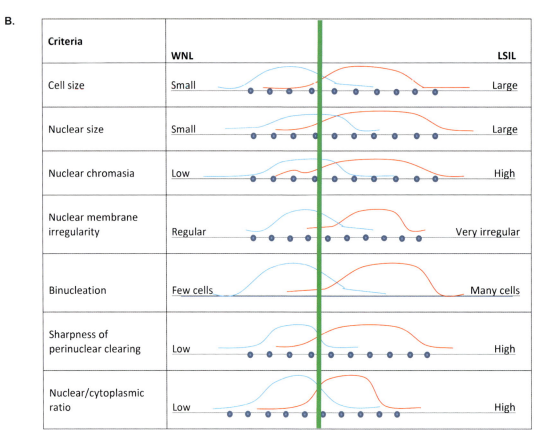

Figure 7-3. A. Pap test low-grade squamous intraepithelial lesion (LSIL) pattern spectrum for an expert pathologist. The black Xs show a "classic" case (every criterion is at the median frequency distribution). Patient VK's Pap test criteria are shown by the red Xs. B. Expert's within normal limits (WNL) LSIL criteria comparison.

Diagnostic Errors and Cognitive Bias

Table 7-4. Examples of Cognitive Heuristics

Type of Heuristic	Description
Availability	A mental shortcut that occurs when individuals make judgments about the probability of events by the availability or ease with which examples come to mind. Imagine that a pathologist examines a thyroidectomy specimen from a 35-year-old woman who had a fine-needle aspiration diagnosed as follicular neoplasm. The pathologist identifies a pattern of numerous, cleared nuclei, in the absence of papillary fragments. The pathologist recalls multiple examples of similar cases that were diagnosed as papillary carcinoma and makes the identical diagnosis (papillary carcinoma) on this specimen.
Representative	A mental shortcut that occurs when individuals make judgments about the probability of events under uncertainty. Imagine that a pathologist examines a clean-catch urine cytology slide, which contains cells displaying highly atypical features (pattern uncertain for malignancy). The pathologist examines the clinical history and determines that the patient is 35 years old and presented with renal colic, and a renal stone from the same patient also was received in the laboratory. The pathologist makes a benign diagnosis because this pattern is "representative" of lithiasis cytology and the patient is young.
Gaze	A mental shortcut that occurs when directing motion to achieve a goal using one main variable—an example is catching a ball. Imagine that a pathologist examines a lung lobectomy specimen from a 67-year-old man who was a smoker and who has a prior bronchial biopsy diagnosis of atypical. The pathologist identifies a large, walled-off area of necrotic debris, but no tumor. The pathologist entirely focuses on the necrosis in the belief that a malignancy is most likely present and has tissue from the entire necrotic area submitted. The pathologist eventually finds a few viable nests of malignant-appearing squamous cells and makes a diagnosis of squamous cell carcinoma.
Anchoring	A mental shortcut to rely heavily (anchor) on the immediate information when making a decision. Imagine that a pathologist examines a liver core specimen from a 62-year-old woman who previously has been diagnosed with metastatic adenocarcinoma. The pathologist quickly examines slides from the core biopsy specimen, identifies malignant cells, and makes the diagnosis of metastatic adenocarcinoma, based on the slide appearance and clinical history.
Effort	A rule of thumb in which the quality or worth of an objective is determined from the perceived amount of effort that goes into producing that objective—if the goal is of lower importance, then the amount of effort is lower. Imagine that a pathologist is provided a larger than normal number of cases, including many biopsies and a few cases that are presumed to be benign (eg, two hernia sacs and a reduction mammoplasty). The pathologist spends most of the day examining the biopsy specimens, because there is a greater likelihood that these specimens may have critical or important information. At the end of the day, the pathologist quickly examines the other specimens and renders benign diagnoses.

Cognitive Strategies in Pattern Recognition

In the first stages of learning the practice of pattern recognition, a novice pathologist examines a slide slowly and carefully to identify criteria and patterns. As a pathologist becomes more experienced, the criteria and patterns are identified more rapidly. The experienced pathologist practices a process of pattern recognition that involves the use of a cognitive heuristic or a mental shortcut that associates the criteria and pattern with a specific disease. Heuristics are simple, efficient rules that explain how people make decisions, come to judgments, and solve problems, typically when facing complex problems or incomplete information.

Heuristic strategies lessen the cognitive load of decision making and are derived from experience with similar problems.[29,30] Heuristics reduce the complexity of clinical judgments in health care. Examples of heuristics are reported in Table 7-4.

Kahneman[31] was awarded a Nobel Prize for his study of cognition and described two cognitive processes: *slow thinking* and *fast thinking*. Slow thinking consists of a rational, deliberate, methodical, and logical process of cognition. Novices practice slow thinking as they learn the process of recognizing criteria and patterns and associating these patterns with specific diseases. Fast thinking is the rapid process of quickly making associations, which all people use most of the time, each day. For example, experienced drivers generally use fast thinking as they drive to and from home each day; driving is a rote process, which does not require deliberate thinking of when and where to turn. Fast thinking employs the use of heuristics, and slow thinking involves delving into the complexity of the problem.

Pathologists use both fast and slow thinking. Experienced pathologists generally build their mental maps using slow thinking but use fast thinking as they examine their daily batch of patient specimens. If experienced pathologists encounter a challenging patient specimen, they may move from fast thinking to slow thinking and more rationally analyze the criteria and patterns of a case. In such a case, they may recognize that the pattern they see does not readily correspond to their mental map for a specific disease and that they need to think more carefully about the information before rendering a definitive diagnosis. Trainees use slow thinking to look at individual cases as they build their mental maps of knowledge.

Interpretive (Diagnostic) Error

An amazing aspect of pathologist pattern recognition practice is the remarkably high frequency of its success and the central role it plays in the diagnostic and screening aspects of medical care. However, because pattern recognition practice is subjective and is based on individual skills and abilities, the practice is limited in several regards. Several of these limitations are outlined below.

Lack of Standardization in Disease Mental Maps

Pathologist disease mental maps are individually and subjectively invented and consequently are subject to variability, which is based on a large number of factors, such as skill, experience, training, case volume, case type, inherent presence of artifacts, internal psychological state, etc. Intuitively, pathologists recognize internal and external differences in how they diagnose specific specimen types as compared with this process of other pathologists. Individual pathologist mental maps may even vary day to day.

An example of this variability is shown in Figure 7-4, A, which depicts a comparative disease pattern spectrum of two expert pathologists for the Pap test diagnoses of WNL and LSIL. The threshold difference is shown in Figure 7-4, B; in this example, expert 1 has a lower threshold for diagnosing LSIL compared with expert 2. It is important to note that this disagreement is fundamental in how the two experts approach the case, using a similar pattern recognition strategy. One difference lies in the processing of the sensory information and linking the pattern to different mental maps. Biases (discussed below) probably contribute to the differences.

The lack of standardization is perhaps the largest component cause of the lack of pathologist agreement detected in secondary review activities. A number of system factors contribute to the lack of standardization, including pathologist practice isolation; the lack of comparative diagnostic outcome data; the inability to maintain individual, firm mental maps; variability in case appearance; and the plateauing of skill sets.

The processes involved in inventing the mental maps (ie, assimilating the knowledge forming the mental map) are highly subject to variability because the steps of assessing stimuli, breaking down and processing the components, memory, and so forth are not performed in a standard manner. Some of the challenges include the following:

- Rank ordering the importance of criteria
- Objectively assessing the frequency of criteria
- Weighing the cutoff of criteria that separate two diseases
- Developing a knowledge bank of all major and minor criteria
- Lacking sufficient experience in assessing the criteria for some diseases or disease variants
- Lacking sufficient experience of how artifacts affect disease representativeness

The lack of standardized work is a system methods process issue because individuals, and even large groups of pathologists, are unable to standardize all diagnostic criteria. Our current repository of mental map knowledge lies in the minds of expert pathologists and is often depicted in fixed formats, such as textbooks or photomicrographs, which demonstrate template, prototype, unusual, or mimic cases. Practice knowledge comes from experiencing the spectrum of variety.

Cognitive Bias

A cognitive bias is a systematic pattern of deviation from the norm or rationality in judgment, whereby inferences may be drawn in an illogical fashion. Individuals create their own subjective reality based on their processing of the sensory stimuli.

As mentioned earlier, heuristics are fast-thinking cognitive shortcuts that allow pathologists to make the leap or association from the recognized pattern to diagnosis. Cognitive biases are slips in the fast-thinking process as an incorrect heuristic is used to achieve a goal of making a diagnosis. This slip often is consciously unrecognized and may be secondary to a number of latent factors. In many cases, more than one bias is at play. Examples of cognitive biases are shown in Table 7-5.

It is important to remember that a cognitive bias does not necessarily result in an error, although it changes the frame of decision making. Cognitive biases limit the more thorough investigation of the issue

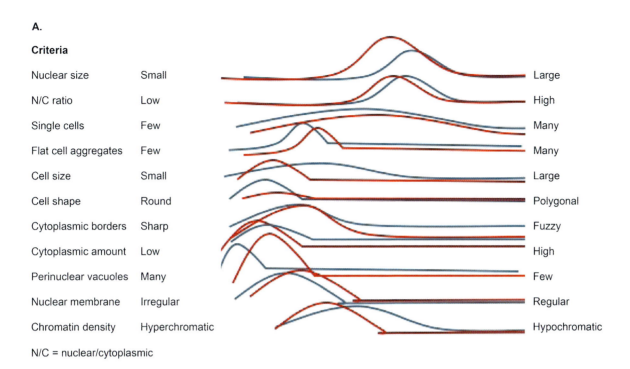

Figure 7-4. A. Pap test low-grade squamous intraepithelial lesion (LSIL) pattern spectrum for expert 1 (red) and 2 (blue). B. Expert 1's (green) and 2's (blue) within normal limits (WNL) LSIL criteria threshold.

and do not involve consideration of a broader range of factors. A challenge in thinking is recognizing the biases that are affecting decision making. The classic example is the blind-spot bias, in which an individual thinks he is less biased than other people.

Diagnostic Errors and Cognitive Bias

Table 7-5. Examples of Cognitive Biases

Bias	Definition	Example
Anchoring	The tendency to rely too heavily (to "anchor") on one trait, past reference, or piece of information when making decisions	A pathologist makes the diagnosis of a malignant melanoma on a lymph node biopsy specimen based on the fact that the patient has a history of malignant melanoma. The pathologist does not include other malignancies that may appear similar (eg, carcinomas, lymphoma, other sarcomas) in the differential diagnosis.
Recency	The tendency to weigh recent events more than earlier events	On the same day, a pathologist makes the diagnosis of cervical intraepithelial neoplasia 3 (CIN III) on biopsy specimens of three different patients. A pathologist makes the same diagnosis on another patient and does not exclude other lesions that may mimic the appearance of CIN III.
Subjective validation	The perception that something is true if an individual's belief demands it to be true	A pathologist examines a challenging lung case and, after performing an extensive immunohistochemical workup, makes a diagnosis of metastatic renal cell carcinoma. The pathologist shows the case to a colleague, who disagrees with the diagnosis. The original pathologist strongly believes that his original diagnosis is correct (because he spent a lot of time on the case) and does not perform any further investigations.
Availability heuristic	Estimating what is more likely by what is more available in memory, which is biased toward vivid, unusual, or emotionally charged examples	A pathologist examines a breast biopsy specimen from a 65-year-old woman. The tissue sections appear very fragmented and admixed with blood. The pathologist vividly remembers a similar-appearing specimen that she diagnosed as malignant. Follow-up of that specimen showed a benign lesion, and, on review, the original core sections showed considerable artifact that limited interpretation. The pathologist experienced tremendous guilt from this event. The pathologist provides an indeterminate diagnosis on the current specimen, even though she believes the specimen is malignant.
Bandwagon	The tendency to do (or believe) things because many other people do (or believe) the same—a bias related to groupthink and herd behavior	A junior pathologist who recently completed a fellowship in soft tissue pathology brings a soft tissue core biopsy to a consensus conference. The most experienced and senior pathologist makes a different diagnosis than that of the junior pathologist. Other pathologists agree. The junior pathologist automatically changes the diagnosis to agree.
Confirmation	The tendency to search for or interpret information in a way that confirms one's preconceptions	A pathologist examines slides from a lung cancer specimen and thinks the tumor is a primary adenocarcinoma. The pathologist orders a limited panel of immunohistochemical studies (cytokeratin 7, thyroid transcription factor-1 [TTF-1], and napsin A), all of which are nonreactive in the tumor cells. The pathologist interprets the specimen as an example of a primary lung adenocarcinoma and that studies did not work in this specific specimen.

Cognitive biases often are described as occurring on the basis of an individual case, although biases may also affect how mental maps are developed. For example, if a pathologist overdiagnoses a lung cancer specimen, future cases may result in the use of more stringent criteria (as the mental map changed), based on a bias of do no harm.

External and internal factors may be related to bias, although there has been little study of these factors in the field of anatomic pathology. For example, biases may be affected by training, emotional state, hectic nature of the work environment, knowledge, specimen artifact, experience, and so forth.

Table 7-5. Examples of Cognitive Biases (continued)		
Bias	Definition	Example
Hindsight	The tendency to see past events as being predictable at the time those events happened	A woman is diagnosed as having an invasive squamous cell carcinoma of the cervix. One year previously, the woman had a Pap test that was interpreted as within normal limits by a cytotechnologist; and, as part of a quality control process, the slide had already been reviewed by a senior cytotechnologist, who concurred with the original diagnosis. In performing cytologic-histologic correlation, a pathologist reviews the Pap test, knowing that the woman has cancer, and finds two locations in which a few cells of high-grade squamous intraepithelial lesion (HSIL) are probably present. The pathologist classifies the Pap test as a screening error.
Clustering illusion	The tendency to see patterns where none exist	A pathologist examines an inflamed cervical biopsy specimen that definitively shows CIN III. The pathologist also sees a pattern of "definitive" desmoplasia around a few deep tumor nests and makes the interpretation of an invasive malignancy. On a loop electrosurgical excision procedure (LEEP) specimen, invasive tumor is not seen, and multiple areas of inflamed, reactive, fibrous tissue are seen without any tumor. On review of the original tumor, the sign-out pathologist still sees the pattern of desmoplasia, even though colleagues disagree.
Do no harm	Judgment based on reducing risk of major harm	A pathologist examines a lung fine-needle aspiration specimen from a 49-year-old patient and thinks that the specimen is malignant. However, because the patient is young and a positive diagnosis would lead to definitive treatment, the pathologist prefers to reduce the risk of major harm (ie, unnecessary lobectomy) and makes the diagnosis of "atypical, carcinoma not excluded."
Information	The tendency to seek information even when it cannot affect action	A patient presents to a hospital in a terminal state and by radiologic imaging is found to have widespread metastatic cancer. On light microscopy, a punch biopsy specimen of a skin lesion shows a poorly differentiated malignancy. The pathologist orders an initial immunohistochemical panel that shows reactivity for vimentin only. The pathologist orders an additional 25 immunohistochemical studies to further characterize the lesion.

Mitigation and Improving Diagnostic Safety

The fields of both Safety I and Safety II provide important data in improving current anatomic pathology patient safety.

In the study of medical error (Safety I), investigators have shown that the current system environment is associated with a number of root causes that contribute to cognitive error. As has been mentioned throughout this chapter, these factors generally contribute to variability in process, and high levels of variability are associated with higher frequency of errors.

Investigators have used a variety of root cause analysis methods to determine immediate causes and latent factors associated with anatomic pathology error. A major focus of improvement based on Safety I research has been the development of standardized practice, which is often a type of best practice. The development of standardized reporting (eg, the College of American Pathologists cancer protocol templates),[32] standardized diagnoses (eg, the Bethesda System for Reporting Cervical Cytology),[33] and standardized diagnostic criteria are all examples of methods to lower cognitive errors. As Safety I investigators have shown that diagnostic errors are associated with poorly designed systems (eg, hectic environments, lack of training, communication gaps), other improvement methods have focused on these system components.

The study of Safety II or the success of current anatomic pathology systems reveals the conditions and practices that already are going right. These conditions and practices are those of resiliency.[11,34,35] Some characteristics of resilient systems are as follows.

Redundancy: The concept of redundancy already exists in a variety of ways in anatomic pathology practice, the most notable being secondary case review methods. Secondary review may serve as a form of standardizing mental maps of disease (a form of reaching consensus) by integrating the pattern recognition processes of individual pathologists or groups of pathologists. In addition, pre–sign-out (proactive) secondary review for individual cases provides a check on cognitive bias or pathologist slips in the cognitive process. Pathologists may perform secondary review in a number of ways (eg, difficult case, rapid review, targeted by disease or organ), which have different strengths and weaknesses. All forms of secondary review have the potential to improve connections and teamwork, which are forms of social cohesion and trust, which are other characteristics of resilient systems.

Learning: Continuous education is an inherent part of pathologist practice, and groups that foster this component may achieve a higher level of resilience. Some group pathologists implicitly learn from each other through methods of consensus in which pattern recognition processes are implicitly evaluated and improved. This consensus method may be used to standardize group mental maps, and this process improves both diagnostic precision and accuracy. Investigators have indicated that an effective means of reducing cognitive bias is through reference class forecasting, which is performed in three steps[36]:

1. Identify a reference class of similar conditions
2. Establish a probability distribution of a specific parameter being forecast
3. Compare the specific parameter with the reference class distribution to establish the most likely outcome for the parameter

The method of establishing the reference range is similar to the process of a subset of pathology research and learning in which specific criteria (eg, gross morphologic criteria, light microscopic criteria, immunohistochemical criteria) are examined for specific disease and nondisease states. The method of shifting to slow thinking to compare specific criteria with the reference range (mental maps) is a method of reducing bias and learning from individual cases. Pathologists who use this deliberate practice method improve their diagnostic skill and eventually may become experts. Practicing pathologists who are able to perform this shift on an individual case basis demonstrate the learning component of a resilient, deliberate practice.

Diversity: The diversity of group components promotes resiliency by increasing the ability to thrive despite shocks and stresses. Examples of diversity in anatomic pathology practice are the growth of ancillary testing methods (which also contributes to learning and interdependency) and the growth of subspecialty expertise. Pathologist cognitive stresses include examining specimens from patients who have rare diseases or rare presentations of common diseases. The development of national expert panels may assist in specific situations by providing diverse and unique expertise as a form of redundancy for general pathologists.

Modularity (disconnectedness): The practice of anatomic pathology is based on modularity, in which individual groups are nodes within a larger system. A system that fosters the interdependence of these nodes also fosters resiliency. Pathology groups vary in size, complexity, practice type, specialized expertise, and a number of other characteristics, which allow for growth and learning in quality practices. For example, some group characteristics lead to the development of high levels of efficiency, whereas other groups foster processes of patient safety. The more these nodes communicate and share activities (eg, consultations, national meetings, social networking), the more individuals within the groups learn about best practices, including those of improving safety.

Other characteristics of resilient systems include adaptation, stability and security, feedback, openness, preparedness, and good governance. These forms of resiliency may be facilitated to improve safety culture within laboratories.

References

1. Taylor FW. *The Principles of Scientific Management.* Eastford, CT: Martino Publishing; 2013.
2. Gartman D. *From Autos to Architecture: Fordism and Architecture Aesthetics in the Twentieth Century.* New York, NY: Princeton Architectural Press; 2009.
3. Oakland JS. *Total Quality Management and Operational Excellence: Text with Cases.* 4th ed. New York, NY: Routledge, Taylor and Francis Group; 2014.
4. Liker JK. *The Toyota Way: 14 Management Principles from the World's Greatest Manufacturer.* New York, NY: McGraw-Hill; 2004.
5. Spear S, Bowen K. *Decoding the DNA of the Toyota Production System.* Boston, MA: Harvard Business Press; 1999.
6. Institute of Medicine. *Envisioning the National Health Care Quality Report.* Washington, DC: National Academy Press; 2001.

7. Rycroft-Malone J, Seers K, Chandler J, et al. The role of evidence, context, and facilitation in an implementation trial: implications for the development of the PARIHS framework. *Implement Sci.* 2013;8:28.
8. Matlin MW. *Cognition.* 8th ed. Hoboken, NJ: John Wiley & Sons, Inc; 2012.
9. Michelon P. What are Cognitive Abilities and Skills, and How to Boost Them? Sharp Brains. http://sharpbrains.com/blog/2006/12/18/what-are-cognitive-abilities/. December 18, 2006. Accessed January 3, 2016.
10. Kohn LT, Corrigan JM, Donaldson MS, eds; Committee on Quality of Health Care in America; Institute of Medicine. *To Err is Human: Building a Safer Health System.* Washington, DC: National Academy Press; 2000.
11. Hollnagel E. *Safety-I and Safety-II: The Past and Future of Safety Management.* Burlington, VT: Ashgate Publishing Company; 2014.
12. Raab SS, Grzybicki DM, Janosky JE, et al. Clinical impact and frequency of anatomic pathology errors in cancer diagnoses. *Cancer.* 2005;104(10):2205-2213.
13. Nakhleh RE, Nosé V, Colasacco C, et al. Interpretive diagnostic error reduction in surgical pathology and cytology: guideline from the College of American Pathologists Pathology and Laboratory Quality Center and the Association of Directors of Anatomic and Surgical Pathology. *Arch Pathol Lab Med.* 2016;140:29-40.
14. Raab SS, Grzybicki DM. Quality in cancer diagnosis. *CA Cancer J Clin.* 2010;60:139-165.
15. Wechsler J, Bastuji-Garin S, Spatz A, et al. Reliability of the histopathologic diagnosis of malignant melanoma in childhood. *Arch Dermatol.* 2002;138:625-628.
16. Raab SS, Meier FA, Zarbo RJ, et al. The "Big Dog" effect: variability in assessing the causes of error in diagnoses of patients with lung cancer. *J Clin Oncol.* 2006;24(18):2808-2814.
17. Reason J. *Human Error.* United Kingdom: Cambridge University Press; 1990.
18. Sternberg RJ. *Cognitive Psychology.* 6th ed. Belmont, CA; Wadsworth Publishing; 2011.
19. Norman DA. *The Design of Everyday Things.* New York, NY: Basic Books; 2013.
20. Shappell SA, Wiegmann DA. *The Human Factors Analysis Classification Scheme – HFACS.* Washington, DC: Office of Aviation Medicine; 2000.
21. Battles JB, Kaplan HS, Van der Schaaf TW, Shea CE. The attributes of medical event-reporting systems: experience with a prototype medical event reporting system for transfusion medicine. *Arch Pathol Lab Med.* 1998;122:231-238.
22. Raab SS, Vrbin CM, Grzybicki DM, et al. Errors in thyroid gland fine needle aspiration. *Am J Clin Pathol.* 2005;125(6):873-882.
23. Chang A, Schyve PM, Croteau RJ, O'Leary DS, Loeb JM. The JCAHO patient safety event taxonomy: a standardized terminology and classification schema for near misses and adverse events. *Int J Qual Health Care.* 2005;17(2):95-105.
24. Margolis H. *Patterns, Thinking, and Cognition: A Theory of Judgment.* Chicago, IL: The University of Chicago Press; 1987.
25. Corrigan MS. *Pattern Recognition in Biology.* New York, NY: Nova Science Publishers; 2007.
26. Yin PY. *Pattern Recognition Techniques, Technology and Applications.* Rijeka, Croatia: InTech Publishers; 2008.
27. Brunelli R. *Template Matching Techniques in Computer Vision: Theory and Practice.* Hoboken, NJ: John Wiley & Sons, Inc; 2009.
28. Biederman I. Recognition-by-components: a theory of human image understanding. *Psychol Rev.* 1987;94(2):115-147.
29. Kahneman D, Slovic P, Tversky A. *Judgment Under Uncertainty.* New York, NY: Cambridge University Press; 1999.
30. Gilovich T, Griffin D, Kahneman D. *Heuristics and Biases: The Psychology of Intuitive Judgment.* New York, NY: Cambridge University Press; 2002.
31. Kahneman D. *Thinking, Fast and Slow.* New York, NY: Farrar, Straus and Giroux; 2013.
32. Cancer Protocol Templates. College of American Pathologists. http://www.cap.org/web/oracle/webcenter/portalapp/pagehierarchy/cancer_protocol_templates.jspx?_adf.ctrl-state=5wjgyrt8z_9&_afrLoop=999023182296123#!. Accessed February 23, 2017.
33. Nayar R, Wilbur DC. *The Bethesda System for Reporting Cervical Cytology.* 3rd ed. New York, NY: Springer; 2015.
34. Zolli A. *Resilience: Why Things Bounce Back.* New York, NY: Simon and Schuster; 2012.
35. Hollnagel E, Woods DD, Leveson N. *Resilience Engineering: Concepts and Precepts.* Burlington, VT: Ashgate Publishing Limited; 2006.
36. Kahneman D, Tversky A. Intuitive prediction: biases and corrective procedures. In: Makridakis S, Wheelwright SC, eds. *Studies in the Management Sciences: Forecasting.* Vol. 12. Amsterdam, Netherlands: North Holland Publishing Company; 1979.

8

Building High-Reliability Teams in the Laboratory

Nicole D. Riddle, MD

Introduction

Patient care has undergone much change in the past several decades. Today, doctors regularly work longer hours, see more patients, and process more cases than did their mentors in the early years of their careers. In addition, as a whole, patients today have more interest in their health care and much more involvement in making decisions about their health care and treatment. Also, easy access to the Internet provides increased information (sometimes correct, sometimes not) to most people. Furthermore, we live in a society where mistakes are not "allowed," doctors have to be perfect, and (too) many people are looking for a way to capitalize on possible or perceived errors. The health care environment is changing drastically, caustic at times, and is something we need to adapt to and help mold for the future of medicine. In this chapter, the goal is to learn more about high-reliability organizations (HROs), how they pertain to health care (and specifically to the laboratory), and how effective team building can help us achieve them. Because this is a relatively new concept and little-researched area, until very recently there was a relative dearth of literature available, and most of the literature consists of reviews and re-reviews or reports of small in-house projects; in addition, articles pertaining to the laboratory have been especially lacking despite the importance of HROs to the hospital system. Just recently, the laboratory did come into view in the Institute of Medicine (IOM) update on patient safety and has been well elucidated for the practicing pathologist in a recent article by Laposata and Cohen.[1] Although many of the examples come from the general health care field, the concepts are translatable to the laboratory setting and will ultimately help achieve the most important goal: safe, effective, efficient patient care.

Background

The 2000 IOM report, *To Err is Human: Building A Safer Health System,* claimed that between 44,000 and 98,000 people died each year in hospitals as a result of medical errors.[2] However, in 2013 a review was released in the *Journal of Patient Safety* that claimed that up to 400,000 people die annually from preventable hospital errors, putting medical errors as the third leading cause of death in the United States.[3] Information websites such as Hospital Safety Score have claimed this further underscores the need for patients to protect themselves and their families from harm and for hospitals to make patient safety a priority.[4] And indeed, Leapfrog, an independent, national, nonprofit organization that rates more than 2500 hospitals with an alphabetical (A-F) score, is an advocate for patient safety nationwide. In 2013, the CEO of Leapfrog was quoted as saying, "A number of hospitals have improved by one or even two grades, indicating hospitals are taking steps toward safer practices, but these efforts aren't enough."[4] And anecdotal stories and individual project research has shown that many hospitals are making headway in addressing and preventing errors, accidents, injuries, and/or infections that cause patient harm, but, unfortunately, the overall progress is slow.

In fact, 3 years later, as this chapter is being written, numerous news outlets have latched on to this information recently published again in *The BMJ* (formerly the *British Medical Journal*) and have started reporting that patients should possibly be concerned if they or a loved one needs hospital-based care.[5-8] Dr. Makary,[9] a professor of surgery from Johns Hopkins University, is quoted as saying, "It boils down to people dying from the care that they receive rather than the disease for which they are seeking care." And *Consumer Reports* has almost a dozen articles aimed at patients with such titles as "Survive Your Hospital Stay"[10] and "What You Don't Know About Your Doctor Could Hurt You."[11]

With new and ever-increasing dissemination of patient safety information (or lack thereof) and our own increased knowledge that these problems exist, it is time that we, as medical professionals, seriously address the weak points in the health care system and make changes to policies and procedures to improve the process.

What Is a High-Reliability Organization and Why Are They Important?

Background

Most health care workers want to do what is best for their patients in the best way possible. The 2000 IOM report recommended the following four-tier approach to improving patient safety:

- Establish a national focus to create leadership, research, tools, and protocols to enhance the knowledge base about safety.
- Identify and learn from errors by developing a nationwide, public, mandatory reporting system and by encouraging health care organizations and practitioners to develop and participate in voluntary reporting systems.
- Raise performance standards and expectations for improvement in safety through the actions of oversight organizations, professional groups, and group purchases of health care.
- Implement safety systems in health care organizations to ensure safe practices at the delivery level.

A 2001 follow-up IOM report, *Crossing the Quality Chasm: A New Health System for the 21st Century,* suggested six aims (health care needs to be safe, effective, patient-centered, timely, efficient, and equitable) and the following 10 rules for redesign of the health care landscape[12]:

- Care is based on continuous, healing relationships.
- Care is customized according to patient needs and values.
- The patient is the source of control.
- Knowledge is shared and information flows freely.
- Decision making is evidence based.
- Safety is a system property.
- Transparency is necessary.
- Needs are anticipated.
- Waste is continuously decreased.
- Cooperation among clinicians is a priority.

The report also suggested four main areas in which changing the structure and process of the health care environment need to occur, as follows:

- Applying evidence to health care delivery
- Using information technology
- Aligning payment policies with quality improvement
- Preparing the workforce

High-Reliability Health Care

High-reliability organizations are not a new concept in general. They have been around from the turn of the 20th century and continue to operate under the assumption that perfection is never achieved and improvements can always be made. Regarding its application to medicine, it primarily was spurred by the IOM's report, *To Err Is Human.*[2] It was this report that really brought to the public eye the number of preventable deaths that occur in hospitals due entirely or in part to a health care mistake. In the article, they defined a medical error as "the failure of a planned action to be completed as intended or the use of a wrong plan to achieve an aim." They list among the other problems (surgical injuries, falls, burns, pressure ulcers, etc) improper transfusions and mistaken patient identities. These are two areas where the laboratory is greatly involved and instances where, although we might not have been mentioned directly, the laboratory is an integral part of fixing the problem.

The Definition of a High-Reliability Organization

The term *high-reliability* refers to the ability of a complex, high-risk industry to go extended periods of time without significant incidents.[13] Examples include the airline industry, amusement theme parks, and nuclear power plants. In order to achieve this level of reliability, these organizations welcome—and even reward—identification of errors and near-misses for the information that can be gleaned from analysis of what occurred before the event. They create an environment ("collective mindfulness") in which all those involved look for and report even small problems or possible unsafe conditions early enough that they are easy to fix and hopefully before they pose a substantial risk (ie, a "near-miss").[14] It is this environment that, although most of us will agree is a good thing, is exceedingly hard to achieve in medicine (see "Barriers to Effective Teamwork and Communication," below, for more explanation).

According to the book *Managing the Unexpected* by Weick and Sutcliffe,[14] HROs have the following five characteristics:

- **Preoccupation with failure:** Never being satisfied there has not been an accident for many months or years; always being aware of the smallest signal that a safety issue may be developing
- **Reluctance to simplify their observations:** Being able to identify often-subtle clues that could make the difference between prevention and early or late recognition
- **Sensitivity to operations:** Recognizing that the earliest indicators of performance threats typically appear in small changes in operations
- **Commitment to resilience:** Recognizing that despite all of their best efforts, errors will still occur
- **Deference to expertise:** Having mechanisms to identify and utilize the individual best suited to manage the new threat situation, no matter what their hierarchical status

Building on these defining characteristics, several authors have argued that if the health care industry could adopt these methods and paradigms of other industry HROs, systemwide improvements in patient safety and health care outcomes would follow.[14,15] Indeed, harm to patients is often the outcome of a cascade of missteps arising from a variety of processes, involving multiple people, and ultimately ending at the patient's bedside.[16] A huge step in becoming a high-reliability health care system—and thereby preventing medical error and decreasing patient harm—is to require improved communication among all health care professionals and utilize teamwork to achieve this goal.

High Reliability by Design

Historically, *organization design* referred to the decomposition of an organization into subparts and then integrating the subparts together to support the strategy and achieve organizational goals. This often includes deciding what an organization will do for itself rather than purchase from others, dividing tasks and assigning roles, choosing appropriate technologies, and establishing and enforcing policies and procedures. In the hospital setting, organization design includes such examples as whether it is public or private, is part of a larger health care system or stand alone, has an emergency department and what level of care is provided, has research interests and/or medical school affiliation, and has in-house or outsourced billing. All of these aspects of the hospital design will affect the laboratory itself and the pathologists who work there. And these concepts can be applied to any laboratory setting, whether it is a small stand-alone laboratory or a large-scale industry.

In 2006, Carroll and Rudolph[17] adapted the theory of organizational design to health care. They approached organizational design with the assumption that they are ever growing, changing, and evolving, as well as being at different stages and having different immediate and future needs. Therefore, no one single design is best for all organizations or even for the same organization at different times; however, they described four stages of redesign and the typical challenges faced in each stage. An awareness of these concepts can aid in accomplishing each institution's unique needs and desires.

The first stage is the *local stage*, where individuals or groups have their own skill sets and ways of dealing with issues. Each hospital department has its own work practices, needs, wants, and constraints. Most of us are astutely aware of the differing opinions between what the surgery department wants and what the laboratory can safely and cost effectively provide. This stage can also be applied to individual physicians, who may feel health care is not a team endeavor (have to do everything themselves) and deny their own vulnerability (eg, working long hours without sleep).[18]

Although local autonomy has some strengths (fostering specialization, innovation, and improvisation), it also leads to the "shame and blame" mentality found among many health care institutions where professionals who require or desire help are seen as not being up to the challenge.[19] We are all keenly aware that physicians do not like to ask for help, nor do they react well to someone telling them how to practice medicine. During the local stage, an organization must be aware of these challenges and use the strengths and experience of the individuals as well as health care professional expertise/specialization to support improvisation and innovation for patient safety. Health care professionals need to be encouraged to appreciate new knowledge and place the patient's well-being at the forefront.

The second stage is the *control stage*, where there is tension between standardization and innovation. How does an organization retain the benefits of control while also addressing novel problems or capitalizing on new opportunities that do not fit into existing procedures? Calling for more standardization and efficiency, which further reduces resources for innovation and quality improvement, is particularly challenging when competition is driving down profit margins. Some aspects of health care thrive in the control stage, where strict policies help us move toward improved patient safety. For example, strict handwashing rules that can be monitored, rewarded, and punished have reduced nosocomial infections. Also, strict checking of patient identification using two or more identifiers and bedside hemolysis checks have decreased the incidence of transfusion-related incidents. But in all of these areas, compliance is not 100%, errors still happen, and being "lean" has caused health care workers to be overworked and rushed. However, too much emphasis on the control stage can lead a health care organization to ignore or discount new information and can bring a false sense of reliability and safety.

The *open stage* is where there are ample opportunities for conversations between cross-functional teams to allow for diverse viewpoints, possible exchanges of personnel, encouragement of participation and mutual respect regardless of hierarchical position, and experimentation with new practices. Organizations operating in the control stage often view those in the open stage as unproductive and illegitimate, and vice versa; however, there are elements that support reliability within the open stage, such as "heedful interrelating," where people attend to each other's concerns and ideas, rely upon and draw out other's specialized knowledge, and respect and value unique perspectives.[20] Here, multiple perspectives are valued, emotions and conflicts are acknowledged and managed appropriately, and trust is fostered across all levels and teams. Cooperation across traditional boundaries is crucial, and those typically considered at the top of the pyramid (eg, surgeons/physicians) must allow themselves to become a partner rather than a dictator[21,22] (see more on this in "Achieving High-Reliability Teams" below). Challenges to this stage include the cost of experimentation—because performance usually declines while new things are tried—and maintaining safe control while learning new things. Also, there are often uneven rates of progress regarding openness, which may lead to interpersonal or interdepartmental conflict.

The final stage is the *deep stage*, which integrates local, control, and open stage practices into systems thinking. *Systems thinking* is a discipline/framework that includes specific tools and techniques that allows health care organizations to perceive interrelationships underlying situations or events and therefore identify short-term and long-term patterns of change. There are several challenges to this stage of reliability. Complex interdependencies among services mean the origins of problems are often obscure, and obvious solutions may not address the problem; also, well-intentioned actions (or quick fixes) may help in the short-term but create other unintended issues.[23] In addition, if a health care organization is successful in obtaining and maintaining this stage, it usually is a result of maintaining some financial "slack" and personnel resources to reflect on and investigate standard operating procedures. As mentioned briefly in the control stage, being lean leads to cost pressures that may lead to reductions in these resources. Effective elements to address these challenges require integration of the strong points of each of the previous stages. For example, by valuing multiple perspectives using the open stage, deep stage organizations can then mobilize local expertise to continually redesign and refine standard operating procedures. And systems-thinking skills allow health care organizations to link rational planning and risk analysis of the control stage while heeding interrelating of the open stage all while using local expertise.

The deep stage uses shared representations (process maps, root cause analyses, organization processes and individual mental models about those processes) to enhance attention to interrelationships and possibilities for improvement. By creating opportunities for people to cross-functionally examine problems, shared representations reduce lapses in safety and reliability, which are often generated by unconnected local perspectives and initiatives. A great example comes from a case where staff members were frustrated about phlebotomy delays that lead to delayed discharges, higher costs, and lost revenue.[24] Each individual group (physicians, nurses, phlebotomists, residents, and laboratory managers) defined the problem on the basis of its local perceptions and blamed others for not seeing the "obvious solution." However, when a task force was formed to investigate the situation, it became evident that the phlebotomists' average blood draw time was actually better than the industry average. The problem was more subtle, resulting from timing of rounds in addition to the distribution, but not the number, of phlebotomists. Only by looking at the interdepartmental and temporal interdependencies, and how local "fixes" exacerbated the problem, were they able to initiate changes that led to a steady decrease in length of stay and an increase in revenue.

The Importance of a High-Reliability Team

Health care is extremely complex and multifaceted, and the risks are also extremely high. Yet, studies have shown time and time again how medicine is not reliable. Too many patients experience preventable harm; have inefficient, ineffective, or inaccessible care; or have care that is not aligned with their goals and beliefs. Because of the points mentioned in the "Introduction" and the IOM articles, news coverage, government involvement, and the overall changing health care environment, there has never been more necessity for high-reliability principles to be incorporated into the health care industry. And this need will only increase as molecular testing expands, technology advances, treatment options grow and become more specific, and patient management becomes more complex.

Note: A relatively short and interesting read is the article, "The Stories Clinicians Tell," by Cohen and Stewart,[16] which uses true medical misadventures to highlight specific elements of unreliability (eg, lack of communication and teamwork), thereby identifying opportunities for improvements in patient safety.

What Constitutes Teamwork and How It Is Achieved

The Definition of Teamwork

Teamwork is generally defined as the combined action of a group of people working together to achieve a common goal, especially when effective and efficient. An efficient team can be trained to help each other maximize their job performance and help to make an inviting and productive atmosphere for new team members. It is important to note that a "group" is not a "team." A group is several people working in close proximity to each other, often with the same project in mind, but not necessarily the same goals. Being a team implies working together in agreed-upon ways to achieve a common goal that has been decided upon together. Teams consist of two or more people (five to seven is usually considered optimal, depending on the situation and size of the project; and an odd number is preferred) who have specific skills, defined roles, perform interdependent tasks, and are adaptable to change and "bumps in the road."[25] Teamwork depends on each team member being able to anticipate the needs of others, adjust to each other's actions, and have a shared understanding of how a procedure should happen (eg, knowing the steps in an apheresis procedure).

It is important to note that simply implementing a team structure does not automatically ensure that it will operate effectively. Teamwork is not an automatic consequence of co-locating people (forming a "group") and depends on a willingness to cooperate for a shared goal. Teamwork does not require that team members work together on a permanent basis but rather is sustained by a commitment to a shared goal.[25]

There are numerous theories on the benefits of and how to achieve teamwork. Specifics are mentioned below for reference purposes, but they represent well-established concepts and a vast literature review.

Benefits of Teamwork

Dave Mattson, CEO of Sandler Training, describes six ways in which teamwork benefits the work place[26]:

Fosters creativity and learning: Creativity thrives when brainstorming occurs as a group and prevents stale viewpoints. Also, combining unique perspectives from each team member typically creates more effective solutions.

Blends complementary strengths: Working together lets teammates build on each other's talents. Try to ensure everyone is aware of each person's abilities to allow the best utilization and distribution of efforts.

Builds trust: Trust provides a feeling of safety that allows ideas to emerge and helps team members open up and encourage each other. Open communication is key when working on a team and helps produce effective solutions in difficult projects. Also, when there is trust in a co-worker, there is an established relationship foundation that can endure minor conflict.

Teaches conflict resolution skills: Team members come from varied backgrounds and have different work styles and habits, which may generate resentment that can quickly turn into conflict. By working to resolve these conflicts, team members learn an important skill that will aid them in the future.

Promotes a wider sense of ownership: By tackling obstacles and creating notable work together, team members usually feel fulfilled and proud of their contributions, while feeling more connected to the organization, which leads to loyalty and higher job satisfaction.

Encourages healthy risk-taking behavior: Often, an employee working alone will not want to risk failure of a novel idea and taking the full brunt of the blame. Working with others spreads out the responsibility, often leading to a greater willingness to try new things.

Teamwork in Health Care

It is easy to see how teamwork is critical for a high-reliability health care system. Given the interdisciplinary nature of the work and the necessity of cooperation among the workers who perform it, teamwork is critical for ensuring patient safety. Health care works when professionals (including physicians, nurses, assistants, pharmacists, and technicians) coordinate their activities to deliver safe and efficient patient care. Teams make fewer mistakes than do individuals, especially when each team member knows their responsibilities as well as those of other team members. For example, by performing interdependent tasks (a pathologist making a diagnosis only after the sample is received and properly processed), all while functioning in specific defined roles (pathologist, clinician/nurse, technologist), the team shares the common goal of safe, reliable care.

Achieving High-Reliability Teams

Chassin and Loeb[15] defined a series of incremental changes that hospitals should undertake in order to progress toward high reliability. These include involving the leadership and obtaining their commitment to achieving zero patient harm (see "Getting your Hospital Board on Board," below), actively cultivating a fully functional culture of safety throughout the organization, and using a widespread deployment of highly effective process improvement tools.[15]

Critical Characteristics of Teamwork

Since the turn of the last century, some research has been done to identify skills that define health care team performance. Examples include using simulations to allow multidisciplinary teams (including physicians, nurses, and technicians) to work together to effectively manage a predetermined crisis in a safe environment. These simulations allow team skills to be both taught and practiced, including communication, cooperation and coordination, making inquiries, giving and receiving constructive feedback, proper leadership, maintaining positive group morale, and reevaluating individual and team actions.[25]

Numerous studies describe the core requirements needed by physicians, nurses, and other health care professionals in order to function effectively and efficiently in a wide variety of health care teams. In 2006, Baker et al[25] reviewed the available studies and concluded that there are eight components that are critical to good teamwork (see below). They postulated that these competencies must be possessed by health care professionals so that they can perform effectively in a variety of teams and in a variety of coordinated tasks required in day-to-day practice, as well as in long-term projects. And indeed, numerous studies have shown that teams whose members possess a commitment to these competencies outperform teams whose members do not.[26-29]

These competencies are often refined over time when team members work together on a more permanent basis. And regardless of whether a team has consistent membership or not, when team members use these skills, they are able to perform with high reliability and efficiency.

The components critical to good teamwork are the following:

Team leadership: The ability to direct and coordinate activities of others, assess individual and team performance, plan and organize actions, assign appropriate tasks, and motivate team members, all while establishing a positive atmosphere.

Examples: Facilitating team-based problem solving, providing performance expectations and acceptable interactions, and synchronizing contributions of individual team members.

Mutual performance (situation) monitoring: The ability to develop a common understanding of the team environment and to apply appropriate task strategies in order to accurately monitor individual and team performance.

Examples: Identifying mistakes/lapses in each other's actions and providing appropriate feedback in order to facilitate self-correction.

Mutual support: The ability to anticipate each other's needs through accurate knowledge about individual responsibilities and skills to perform them.

Examples: Having potential "back-up" providers recognizing that there is a workload distribution problem and shifting work responsibilities to underutilized team members.

Adaptability: The ability to adjust strategies on the basis of environmental information through the use of compensatory behavior and reallocations of intrateam resources—altering a course of action in response to changing conditions, whether internal or external to the team.

Examples: Identifying cues that a change has occurred, assigning meaning to that change, and developing a new plan to deal with it; identifying opportunities for improvement and innovation for routine practices; remaining vigilant to changes in both the internal and external team environment.

Shared mental models: An organized knowledge structure of the relationship between the task the team is performing and how the team members will interact.

Examples: Anticipating each team member's needs, identifying changes in the team or task and adjusting strategies as needed.

Communication: The exchange of information between a "sender" and a "receiver, whether it is verbal, written, or visual.

Examples: Following up with team members to assure your message was received, acknowledging that their message was received, and clarifying that the message received was the intended message sent.

Team orientation: The propensity to take another's behavior into account during group interactions and the belief in the importance of team goals over individual desires.

Examples: Taking into account any alternative resolutions provided by all team members and appraising that input to determine what is the best option; and increasing task involvement, information sharing, strategizing, and team goal setting.

Mutual trust: The shared belief that each member will perform his or her role and protect the interests of the team members.

Examples: Information sharing and willingness to admit mistakes and accept feedback.

It is important to note that the above components focus on the individual, rather than on the whole team; in other words, each team member must adhere to these competencies when engaging in a team task, and the competencies are not unique to the team or to the task.

The Structure of a Highly Effective Team

The structure of a highly effective team is the essential element to its overall success. First, an effective team should have a team leader who encourages a high level of collaboration and interdependency by providing the necessary support and structure for the team.[30] The first task is putting together the right people. The leader should focus on the systems and practices in the team, not on the personalities of its members. Team members should be chosen and their tasks assigned with their skills in mind. In general, an effective team will consist of five to eight members, and possibly up to 12 or more if a wide diversity of knowledge and opinions is needed. In addition, the team must have the resources and training required to develop any needed skills to complete their tasks.

Utilizing cross-training increases awareness of all tasks that are interdependent, thus increasing team flexibility and improving response time. It is the team leader's job to ensure that all team members understand the purpose of the group and their role in it, are active toward meeting that purpose and role, and utilize procedures for making decisions and solving problems. A leader does not always have to have a strong, charismatic personality. Although that type of personality can often be very successful at developing teams, it may create passivity or frustration in other members over time, thereby hindering effectiveness.

Second, the quality of the team's work is often dependent on the timeliness and quality of constructive feedback, both from the team leader and from fellow team members. Not only crucial to the overall team's effectiveness, appropriate and timely feedback ensures that goals are met and adjustments or corrections are made quickly to avoid delays. And if feedback is received too late, not only will it probably have little practical value for the task at hand, but then it often ends up feeling like criticism. For the team leader, timely, constructive feedback is a tool used to keep team members on task as well as encouraging them to work together, making the difference between a team that hides mistakes and one that views mistakes as opportunities to improve. If a team utilizes these opportunities, it shows that the team leader has successfully created an environment that promotes communication and problem solving. Also, when people are allowed to take part in creating their own solutions, they are more proactive, engaged, and have greater ownership. Although this is an important part of a team leader's responsibility and something all team members should participate in, specifically designating another person to help share that "burden" can help improve relationships among all team members and help alleviate the "disciplinarian" aspect that can occur.

When a team has poor structure (eg, bad leadership or inappropriate team member skills for the assigned tasks), it can actually create ineffective or negative behaviors as well as impede communication. Although the responsibility for poor team performance lies in the poor structure, often the members are blamed or seen as incompetent. Also, if team members feel like they are competing against one another, they will withhold useful information, thereby impeding the overall progress of the team. Whenever a team has problems, it is the team leader's job to focus on the structure, communication, and trust to assure that the team stays on task. In fact, the most effective team leaders are often not an active member of the team in that they limit their opinions on solutions and focus more on helping others work well together. If the team leader has an agenda of what should be done or how it should be accomplished, their ability to lead effectively will be greatly hindered.

A useful, but not required, element of team structure is a communicator—namely, someone who is responsible for ensuring all members receive the regular communications as described below. Communication should also occur with crucial people outside of the team, especially those who make the ultimate decisions or determine the success of the outcome.

Guidelines for Effective Team Building and Managing

Often, teams are merely a gathering of people with perceived importance and not necessarily those with the best skills for or knowledge of the task at hand, and then the assumption is that they will find a way to successfully work together. But, as described above, teams are most effective when they are carefully structured and team members are picked on the basis of their skills related to the task at hand, not necessarily their hierarchical position. Also, all members need to be equal members of the team and feel free to (respectfully) speak their minds and feel their opinions are valued—the team leader is assigned with assuring this occurs and that the team is effective. The following guidelines may help in developing and supporting a highly effective team.

Contact each team member. Before the first meeting, invite each potential team member to be a part of the team. First, send a memo/email, and then, depending on how well you know the person (their skills, personality), consider meeting in person. Talk about the goals of the project, why the individual was selected, his or her benefit to the organization, the time frame for the team effort, and who will lead the team. Invite the team member to the first meeting.

Carefully plan the first meeting. In the first meeting, discuss the reason why the team was formed and the time frame for the team effort, why each member was selected, each individual's perceived benefit to the organization, who will lead the team, and any changes that have occurred since the individual meetings. In addition, try to reach a consensus of when and where the team will meet to ensure the most participation. If walking the laboratory staff to surgery will have better participation of the surgical staff, consider it. Also, come up with "team ground rules" (eg, no cell phones, mutual respect). Once this information is determined, have it written down and communicated to the members in the agreed-upon method (see below). At the end of the meeting, ask each person to make a public commitment to the team effort. And remember, meetings often fill the time they are allotted; if the team meetings can be 20 to 30 minutes, then schedule them as such. And be sure to start and end on time. Showing respect for others' time and outside responsibilities goes a long way toward effective team building.

Plan team-building activities to support trust and working relationships. In the first or second meeting, have members introduce themselves and come up with an interesting question they can answer about themselves. Farther along in team progress, consider a session when members can voice their concerns and frustrations about their team assignments.

Set clear goals/objectives. There are many ways to design team goals, and as long as the end result is successful and within the time frame expected, the exact mechanism is open for variation based on situational factors and team members' personalities. In fact, as much as possible, input from all team members should be acquired when designing and wording the team goals. A useful acronym to make sure that all of the appropriate components are considered is SMART, which stands for Specific, Measurable, Achievable, Relevant, and Time bound. The goals and specifics should be written and available for review throughout the course of the project/team performance and adjusted as needed as issues and new information arise. An example would be "Within 6 months, develop an efficient and more cost-effective courier system while ensuring integrity of patient specimens."

Define clear and consistent communication mechanisms. Leaders, and, indeed, most people often assume that all group members know what the leader knows. Clear and consistent communication is possibly the most important trait of an effective team. All members should regularly receive information about the team, such as goal reminders, membership changes, progress status, and accomplishments. Communications may be via regular newsletters, status reports, meetings, emails, and/or collaboration tools. The system used should be discussed and agreed upon by all (or most—vote if needed) team members to ensure that the best communication methods are chosen, thereby increasing the chances of successful communication. Also, to ensure effective use of the meeting time; it is good to have a clear agenda set and communicated for each meeting in advance.

Define a procedure to make decisions and solve problems. All teams regularly encounter situations where decisions must be made or problems solved, preferably in a highly effective manner. Often this leads to extended discussion until members become tired and frustrated, and eventually just opt for any action at all, or they resort to accepting the decision of the person with the strongest opinion. In an effective team, members will mutually define a procedure for how decisions will be made. A good procedure will include something to the effect that all solutions/opinions will be heard, calling on each member individually if needed, and then aiming for consensus or holding a vote.

Develop staffing procedures (recruiting, training, organizing, and replacing). Over the course of a longer team project, members may need to move off the team for numerous reasons, possibly requiring a replacement; or new skills may be needed, leading to additional team members being added. When new members are added to a previously established team, an organized, systematic process to get them "up to speed" will show them that the team is well organized and their role is valuable; it will allow them to become an effective member more quickly as well as help build trust between them and previous team members. This becomes even more important if a team member is being replaced under "bad terms." It is important to keep in mind what roles and types of expertise are needed and choose according to plans, not personality. It is also important to ensure that the new member understands his or her purpose, role, next steps, and where to get help.

Identify needs for any additional resources (training, materials, and supplies). Start by analyzing the purpose and goals of the team. What is needed to achieve them? What training might members benefit from that provides a brief overview of the typical stages of team development and includes packets of materials about the team's goals, structure, and process to make decisions. Consider costs directly related to team function above what is expected as part of usual work. How will those funds be obtained and maintained?

Regularly monitor and report status. Many times a team starts out with carefully designed plans but then abandons them when the initial implementation is underway. Or, if the plan is behind schedule, team members may conclude that the project is not successful. Plans and goals may change, but if that occurs it should be done systematically, with new dates and team approval. And updates should be sent in a communication.

Regularly celebrate team members' accomplishments. This is one of the best ways to avoid burnout. Acknowledging their accomplishments rejuvenates and encourages team members to continue to succeed. Otherwise, members may begin to feel as if they are a hamster on a wheel. Look out for small and recurring successes and bring attention to them accordingly.

Stages of Teamwork

While using all of these structural and procedural guidelines, there is a specific path most teams follow on their way to high reliability and performance. Coined in 1965 by psychologist Bruce Tuckman,[31] the stages of the path include "forming, storming, norming, and performing." Tuckman and Jensen[32] later added "adjourning" in 1977 to include the final resolution of the team. These stages are important to know and understand, because by going through them, a team builds trust and finds its way of working together. Although the stages are described in sequential order, not all teams will progress the same way. Sometimes there are team member changes that lead back to forming; or issues may occur during performing that lead to the team reverting back to storming; and sometimes (with a little luck) the team skips from forming to norming. But however the team proceeds through the stages, as long as it ends with performing and successful completion of tasks and goals, all while maintaining mutual respect and a reasonable timetable within the given resources, that is an effective team outcome.

Forming

In this stage, most team members are positive and polite. Some may be anxious, perhaps because they don't fully understand the team goals. Others may be excited about the task ahead. The team leader plays a dominant role in this stage because the members' roles and responsibilities aren't yet clear, and the ground rules have not yet been established. The mission is not yet "owned" by the group, nor is there trust or commitment within the team. This stage can last for some time as people start to work together, get to know one another, and form a history together trying to reach a common goal.

Steps to move from forming to storming include setting the mission/goals, finding ways to build trust, defining a reward system, taking risks, establishing each person's role (including an understanding of the need to move out of the forming stage), and having them decide once and for all if they will remain on the team.

Storming

The storming phase is where roles and responsibilities are articulated, but members begin to push against the previously established boundaries, and some may want to modify the team's mission to fit their needs/wants. This is the stage where many teams fail. Problem solving does not work well yet, subgroups/cliques are formed, there is little team spirit, there are possibly some verbal personal attacks, and anxiety levels are high. Storming often starts when there are conflicting team member work styles. People work in different ways and for all sorts of reasons, but differing work styles can cause people to become frustrated, communication can break down, and tempers can flare. In addition, team members may challenge the team leader's authority or fight for positions or power as their roles are clarified. If there hasn't been clear definition of how the team will work, members may feel overwhelmed by their perceived (or actual) workload. Others may just be uncomfortable with the approach the leader is using (many individuals—perhaps even the team leader—aren't knowledgeable in the ways of an effective team). If a member questions the worth of the team's goal, he or she may resist taking on responsibility. Storming is often the time of highest participation by the loudest members and lowest participation for the quietest.

In order to go from storming to norming, the team leader should actively support and reinforce team behavior, create a positive environment, facilitate group wins by asking for and expecting results, encourage active listening and discussions to help members agree on their roles and responsibilities and buy into the objectives, include everyone in the responsibility to actively set a supportive environment where anyone can call out another's inappropriate pessimism or aggression, request and accept feedback, and try to instill the vision that "we can succeed!"

Norming

It is hoped that the team will eventually, gradually move into the norming stage when people start resolving their differences, build trust, appreciate each other's strengths, and respect the leader's authority. Members now know each other better, and they are able to ask each other for help, provide constructive feedback, and may even socialize outside of the team meetings. There is a stronger commitment to the team goal, and progress is being made. Team confidence is high, commitment has grown, and the leader should actively reinforce appropriate, productive behavior. Remember that there is often some overlap between storming and norming, because as new issues or tasks arise, the team may lapse back into storming behaviors.

To get from norming to performing, the team must maintain the ground rules and agreed-upon procedures, praise and flatter each other, self-evaluate without issue, share leadership on the basis of skills, share rewards and successes as well as responsibility, and, above all, continue having clear, open communication.

Performing

The team has reached the performing stage when their hard work leads to achievement without associated friction while supported by the structures and processes previously set up, and they feel very motivated to continue. There is high pride in the team with much trust, openness, and support. Members have a "We" instead of an "I" approach. The leader should continue to concentrate on encouraging and developing team members and praising the work being done.

Adjourning

Many times we will reach the adjourning stage, whether due to a predetermined fixed timespan or to disbanding through organizational restructuring. Team members who like routine or who have close working relationships with other members may find this stage difficult (hence it is sometimes referred to as mourning). But if the team was effective and successful, the members will feel a sense of accomplishment and be even more high functioning for the next team.

Barriers to Teamwork and Effective Communication

Despite serious and widespread efforts to improve the quality of health care, many patients still suffer preventable harm daily. Hospitals often find improvement difficult to sustain and suffer "project fatigue" due to there being so many problems that need addressing. Also, there are ways that HROs generate and maintain high levels of safety that cannot be directly applied to the health care system.[15] In addition, the presence of doctors themselves makes many of these changes a challenge, particularly when teamwork is involved.[33] However, despite the importance of teamwork in health care, most clinical units continue to function as discrete and separate collections of professionals. This is partially due to the fact that members of these teams are rarely trained together; furthermore, they often come from separate disciplines and diverse educational programs. Fortunately, most of these barriers can be addressed and removed with proper education and continued work. As alluded to below, starting with health care training is the first step to effect this change.

One particular article pertaining to overcoming barriers to effective teamwork describes seven actions to facilitate team communication[34]:

- **Teach effective communication strategies:** Such as Situation, Background, Assessment, and Recommendation (SBAR) handovers; Time Outs; and Structured Interdisciplinary Bedside Rounds (SIBR)
- **Train teams together:** Shown to promote better understanding of others' roles in improving team efficiency
- **Train teams using simulation:** Using debriefings and recordings with playback—seeing how you appear to others can be a powerful motivator
- **Define inclusive teams:** Define as a cohesive team as opposed to a collection of different professionals
- **Create democratic teams:** So all members feel assured of being heard, feel valued and important, and so that trust can be established
- **Support teamwork with protocols and procedures:** To ensure all team members (including the patient, when appropriate) are present and all information is available when important decisions are to be made; examples: Surgical Safety Checklist, Time Out, and Daily Safety Calls
- **Develop an organizational culture supporting health care teams:** Improving communications to decrease inefficiencies and decrease costs due to delays in treatment, waste of resources, and prolonged hospital stays

The above steps are a great way to start to effect change and improve communication and teamwork.

Using Teamwork to Effect Change

As described above, communication failure is a known leading source of adverse events in health care. Numerous independent studies have shown and The Joint Commission has said this for more than 30 years. Several large studies have demonstrated high levels of coordination and improved communication among staff members, and the positive results include reduced morbidity and mortality and increased job retention.[35-37] *Crew resource management* (CRM; originally known as *cockpit resource management*) is the model in which the focus is on safety, efficiency, and morale of the persons working together. And although there are no definitive studies correlating CRM training with enhanced flight safety, the aviation industry generally accepts it, and it is a requirement for all aviation employees.[38]

The Ability of Teams to Influence Across Boundaries

CRM has many translational aspects into health care, namely the application of countermeasures such as briefings, debriefings, standardized communication language and process, workload distribution, fatigue management, inquiry, graded assertiveness, contingency planning, and conflict resolution.[39] And indeed, the Veterans Health Administration has implemented a Medical Team Training (MTT) that is based on CRM principles.[40] The MTT was designed to test two hypotheses: (1) improving patient outcomes and (2) enhancing job satisfaction among health care professionals. To achieve this, they instituted four components: (1) application, preparation, and planning; (2) interactive learning session hosted by the participating Veterans Affairs medical center; (3) implementation of MTT project and follow-up with National Center for Patient Safety faculty; and (4) MTT program evaluation. The results from the multi-institutional nationwide endeavors showed numerous improvements, such as participation of surgical teams in the operating room, more proactive circulating nurses and administration between departments, and less time running around looking for instruments. All of these things and more have improved the quality of patient care and personnel job satisfaction at these institutions, and plans are to expand the program to other hospitals.

Team Huddles and the Use of Teams

Like most things in medicine, processes to improve communication among health care professionals should be standardized to improve efficiency and efficacy. Teams that jointly evaluate a patient, obtain a history, and perform a physical are able to reduce redundancy, save time, and increase both staff and patient satisfaction.[41] In addition, well-functioning, patient-focused, team-based care is associated with increased quality, increased productivity, decreased costs, and improved outcomes.[42] There are numerous tools and strategies to help increase the amount and quality of communication (see below). Two common and well-vetted structured communication methods are huddles and the use of SBAR (situation, background, assessment, and recommendation).[43-45] The Institute for Healthcare Improvement (IHI)[46] and TeamSTEPPS[47] recommend strategies such as huddles and, specifically, SBAR to increase the quality and amount of communication, and indeed this framework has been implemented across the nation as a best practice for information delivery.

Some Common Strategies to Improve Communication

There are numerous resources available for improving communication, including journal articles, books, webinars, and in-person seminars. Below are some common strategies that are often discussed within these different modalities.[34]

Closed-loop communication. This three-step strategy involves the sender directing the instruction to the receiver, using his or her name when possible; the receiver confirming the information as a check on hearing and understanding, and seeking clarification if required; then, the sender verifying that the message was correctly received and interpreted.

Graded assertion. The process by which the sender opens and frames the discussion utilizing escalating concern (Probe, Alert, Challenge, Emergency [PACE]).

Step-back (call-out). The health care professional leading the team steps back and reviews the situation, then calls attention to the team to provide an update of the situation and the plan, and invites suggestions.

Structured handover. The process of using simple templates for summarizing important patient information during handovers.

Structured information transmission. ISBAR—Identify, Situation, Background, Assessment, Recommendation—is a widely used acronym for a strategy to help structure verbal handover or patient referral. The shorter version, SBAR, is also used.

Getting Your Hospital Board on Board

As part of the IHI's 5 Million Lives Campaign, fully engaging governance leadership in quality and safety was the only nonclinical intervention among the 12 recommendations. This is more commonly known as *getting the board on board*.[48-51]

Why It Is Necessary

As hospitals seek to rapidly attain quality health care, boards have the opportunity and the responsibility to make better quality care their top priority. In the past, hospital governance was only viewed as being responsible for the organization's financial health and reputation, but now it must also oversee the mission, strategy, quality, and safety.[49] A well-run board will provide accountability, motivation, and set expectations for high performance and the elimination of harm.[51] And like most aspects of medicine and, indeed, of life, effective change is difficult to accomplish and maintain if those in leadership do not have a vested interest.

How It Can Be Done

The goal for the IHI's getting the board on board was for all hospital boards to undertake the six key governance leadership activities to improve quality and reduce patient harm. At a minimum, boards should spend greater than 25% of each meeting's time discussing quality and safety issues and should, as a full board, meet with at least one patient or family member who sustained serious harm at their institution within the previous year. The six recommendations, described in the sixth and final article by James Conway,[49] are as follows:

Setting aims. Make an explicit, public commitment to reducing harm and increasing measurable quality improvement.

Getting data and hearing stories. Make reviewing progress toward safer care the first agenda item at every board meeting, with an emphasis on transparency and by meeting with patients and/or family members.

Establishing and monitoring system-level measures. Identify a group of organization patient safety measures that are continually updated and are transparent to the organization and patients.

Changing the environment, policies, and cultures. Commit to establishing and maintaining a respectful and fair environment for all people who experience pain and loss due to avoidable harm and adverse outcomes, including patients, family members, and the staff involved.

Learning. Develop a way for the board to learn about how the "best boards in the world" work with executive and medical staff members to reduce harm.

Establishing accountability. Include executive team accountability for clear quality improvement targets.

Getting support from your executive staff and hospital boards can be pivotal in the success of quality health care improvement and achieving high reliability. The discussion here is a primer, and further reading of the references is recommended.

Teaching Teamwork to the Next Generation

Traditional training and education of physicians, nurses, and allied health professionals has historically focused on individual technical skills for proficiency of specific tasks. We have been trained in "silos" (think of the difference between pathologists and surgeons, let alone between physician and nonphysician professionals) and then thrown into a very complex environment that is dependent on multiteam systems where the individuals with their distinct areas of expertise are expected to work together to provide efficient, effective, and safe health care.[25] Attention has recently been turned to how professionals are trained and work together in the complex and ever-changing world of health care, and, to this end, the IOM has recommended the application of CRM to training in health care systems, like what the Veterans Health Administration system has done (see above).[40]

In addition to the traditional separate trainings, medicine is practiced in a system in which roles and levels have been clearly differentiated, and consequences can be severe if the hierarchy is perceived as not being followed. Physicians tend to be at the top of this pyramid (except in cases where administrators pull rank), and treatment tends to be performed by nurses, technicians, and others who are following "orders." This hierarchical system makes coordination and cohesion extremely difficult to achieve, especially if not everyone on the team wishes to subscribe to this new paradigm. There has even been research showing that issues between physicians and nurses in particular can contribute to suboptimal care.[52]

Fortunately, times are changing and so is medical education, albeit slowly. There have been several studies pertaining to training medical students to be more amenable to a team approach to health care, including training medical students and nursing students together.[54-58] These studies show that regardless of which approach is used, simply addressing the concept of teamwork and coordinated care improves communication and patient outcome.[54]

Although fundamentally essential to team building and high-reliability health care, to elaborate further on training is beyond the scope of this chapter. Please refer to chapter 9, *Developing a Patient Safety Curriculum for Resident and Fellow Education,* and the articles referenced in this chapter for more information.

References

1. Laposata M, Cohen M. It's our turn: implications for pathology from the Institute of Medicine's report on diagnostic error. *Arch Pathol Lab Med.* 2016;140(6):505-507.
2. Kohn LT, Corrigan JM, Donaldson MS, eds; Committee on Quality of Health Care in America; Institute of Medicine. *To Err is Human: Building a Safer Health System.* Washington, DC: National Academy Press; 2000.
3. James JT. A new, evidence-based estimate of patient harms associated with hospital care. *J Patient Saf.* 2013;9(3):122-128.
4. Hospital Errors are the Third Leading Cause of Death in U.S., and New Hospital Safety Scores Show Improvements are Too Slow. http://www.hospitalsafetyscore.org/newsroom/display/hospitalerrors-thirdleading-causeofdeathinus-improvementstooslow. Hospital Safety Score. October 23, 2013. Accessed February 8, 2016.
5. Cha AE. Researchers: medical errors now third leading cause of death in United States. https://www.washingtonpost.com/news/to-your-health/wp/2016/05/03/researchers-medical-errors-now-third-leading-cause-of-death-in-united-states/. *The Washington Post.* May 3, 2016. Accessed May 9, 2016.
6. Allen M, Pierce O. Medical errors are no. 3 cause of U.S deaths, researchers say. NPR. http://www.npr.org/sections/health-shots/2016/05/03/476636183/death-certificates-undercount-toll-of-medical-errors. *Shots: Health News from NPR.* May 3, 2016. Accessed May 9, 2016.
7. Frellick M. Medical error is third leading cause of death in US. http://www.medscape.com/viewarticle/862832. *Medscape.* May 3, 2016. Accessed May 9, 2016
8. Rubin R. Medical error is a leading cause of death, but you won't see it on the CDC's list. http://www.forbes.com/sites/ritarubin/2016/05/04/medical-error-is-a-leading-cause-of-death-but-you-wont-see-it-on-the-cdcs-list/#715896bd6378. Forbes. May 4, 2016. Accessed May 9, 2016
9. Makary MA, Daniel M. Medical error—the third leading cause of death in the US. *BMJ.* 2016;353:i2139.
10. Survive your hospital stay. http://www.consumerreports.org/cro/magazine/2014/05/survive-your-hospital-stay/index.htm. *Consumer Reports.* March 2014. Accessed February 8, 2016.

11. Peachman RR. What you don't know about your doctor could hurt you. http://www.consumerreports.org/cro/health/doctors-and-hospitals/what-you-dont-know-about-your-doctor-could-hurt-you/index.htm. *Consumer Reports.* April 2016. Accessed May 9, 2016.
12. Richardson WC, Berwick DM, Bisgard JC, eds; Committee on Quality of Health Care in America; Institute of Medicine. *Crossing the Quality Chasm: A New Health System for the 21st Century.* Washington, DC: National Academy Press; 2001.
13. Dupree ES. High reliability: the path to zero harm. *Joint Commission Healthcare Executive.* 2016;Jan/Feb:66-69.
14. Weick KE, Sutcliffe KM. *Managing the Unexpected.* Hoboken, NJ: Jossey-Bass; 2015.
15. Chassin MR, Loeb JM. High-reliability health care: getting there from here. *Milbank.* 2013;91(3):459-490.
16. Cohen DL, Stewart KO. The stories clinicians tell: achieving high reliability and improving patient safety. *Perm J.* 2016;20(1):85-90.
17. Carroll JS, Rudolph JW. Design of high reliability organizations in health care. *Qual Saf Health Care.* 2006;15(Suppl 1):i4-i9.
18. Kellogg K. Challenging Operations: Changing Interactions, Identities, and Institutions in a Surgical Teaching Hospital [dissertation]. Cambridge, MA: MIT Sloan School of Management; 2005. https://dspace.mit.edu/handle/1721.1/33414. Accessed February 8, 2016.
19. Leape LL. Error in medicine. *JAMA.* 1994;272:1851-1857.
20. Weick KE, Roberts KH. Collective mind in organizations: heedful interrelating on flight decks. *Admin Sci Q.* 1993;38:356-381.
21. Berwick DM, Nolan TW. Physicians as leaders in improving health care. *Ann Intern Med.* 1998;128:289-292.
22. Edmondson A. Disrupted routines: team learning and new technology implementation in hospitals. *Admin Sci Q.* 2002;46:685-716.
23. Sterman J, Repenning N, Kofman F. Unanticipated side effects of successful quality programs: exploring a paradox of organizational improvement. *Manage Sci.* 1997;43:503-521.
24. Quinn TD, Rudolph JW, Fairchild D. Lab turnaround time and delayed discharges: a systems-based action research investigation. Boston, MA: Boston University School of Public Health; Health Services Case Study, 2004.
25. Baker DP, Day R, Salas E. Teamwork as an essential component of high-reliability organizations. *Health Serv Res.* 2006;41(4 pt 2):1576-1598.
26. Mattson D. 6 benefits of teamwork in the workplace. https://www.sandler.com/blog/6-benefits-of-teamwork-in-the-workplace. *Professional Development.* February 19, 2015. Accessed February 8, 2016.
27. Smith-Jentsch KA, Salas E, Baker DP. Training team performance-related assertiveness. *Pers Psych.* 1996;49(4);909-936.
28. Salas E, Burke CS, Bowers CA, Wilson KA. Team training in the skies: does crew resource management (CRM) training work? *Hum Factors.* 2001;43:641-674.
29. O'Shea G, Driskell JE, Goodwin GF, Salas E, Weiss S. *Assessment of Team Competencies: Development and Validation of a Conditional Reasoning Measure of Team Orientation.* Washington, DC: US Army Research Institute for the Behavioral and Social Sciences; 2003.
30. Musselhite C. Building and leading high performance teams. http://www.inc.com/resources/leadership/articles/20070101/musselwhite.html. *Inc.* January 1, 2007. Accessed February 8, 2016.
31. Tuckman B. Developmental sequence in small groups. *Psychol Bull.* 1965;63:384-399.
32. Tuckman B, Jensen M. Stages of small group development. *Group Org Stud.* 1977;2:419-427.
33. Rosenstein AH. The quality and economic impact of disruptive behaviors on clinical outcomes of patient care. *Am J Med Qual.* 2011;26(5):372-379.
34. Weller J, Boyd M, Cumin D. Teams, tribes and patient safety: overcoming barriers to effective teamwork in healthcare. *Postgrad Med J.* 2014;90:149-154.
35. Knaus WA, Draper EA, Wagner DP, Zimmerman JE. An evaluation of outcomes from intensive care in major medical centers. *Ann Intern Med.* 1986;104:410-418.
36. Baggs J, Ryan SA, Phelps CE, Richeson JF, Johnson JE. The association between interdisciplinary collaboration and patient outcomes in a medical intensive care unit. *Heart Lung.* 1992;21:18-24.
37. Shortell SM, Zimmerman JE, Rousseau DM, et al. The performance of intensive care units: does good management make a difference? *Med Care.* 1994;32:508-525.
38. Helmreich R, Wilhelm J. Outcomes of crew resource management training. *Int J Aviat Psychol.* 1991;1(4):287-300.
39. Helmreich RL, Merritt AC. *Culture at Work in Aviation and Medicine: National, Organizational and Professional Influences.* Brookfield, VT: Ashgate Publishing; 2001.
40. Dunn EJ, Mills PD, Neily J, Crittenden MD, Carmack AL, Bagian JP. Medical team training: applying crew resource management in the Veterans Health Administration. *Jt Comm J Qual Patient Saf.* 2007;33(6):317-325.
41. Mazzocato P, Forsberg H, Schwartz U. Team behaviors in emergency care: a qualitative study using behavior analysis of what makes teams work. *Scan J Trauma Resusc Emeg Med.* 2011;19:70-76.
42. Leonard M, Frankel A. Role of effective teamwork and communication in delivering safe, high-quality care. *Mt Sinai J Med.* 2011;78:820-826.
43. Lown B, Manning C. The Schwartz Center Rounds: evaluation of an interdisciplinary approach to enhancing patient-centered communication, teamwork, and provider support. *Acad Med.* 2010;85:1073-1081.
44. Creswick N, Westbrook J, Braithwaite J. Understanding communication networks in the emergency department. *BMC Health Serv Res.* 2009;9:247.
45. Martin HA, Ciurzynski SM. Situation, background, assessment, and recommendation-guided huddles improve communication and teamwork in the emergency department. *J Emerg Nurs.* 2015;41(6):484-488.
46. Institute for Healthcare Improvement. Resources for improvement efforts. http://www.ihi.org/resources/Pages/default.aspx. Accessed May 9, 2016.
47. Agency for Healthcare Research and Quality. TeamSTEPPS. http://teamstepps.ahrq.gov. Accessed May 9, 2016.

48. McCannon CJ, Hackbarth AD, Griffin FA. Miles to go: an introduction to the 5 Million Lives Campaign. *Jt Comm J Qual Patient Saf.* 2007;33:477-484.
49. Conway J. Getting boards on board: engaging governing boards in quality and safety. *Jt Comm J Qual Patient Saf.* 2008;34(4):214-220.
50. 5 Million Lives Campaign. *Getting Started Kit: Governance Leadership "Boards on Board" How-to Guide.* Cambridge, MA: Institute for Healthcare Improvement; 2008.
51. Joshi MS, Hines SC. Getting the board on board: engaging hospital boards in quality and patient safety. *Jt Comm J Qual Patient Saf.* 2006;32:179-187.
52. Knox G E, Simpson K R. Teamwork: the fundamental building block of high-reliability organizations and patient safety. In: Youngberg BJ, Hatlie MJ, eds. *Patient Safety Handbook.* Boston, MA: Jones and Bartlett; 2004:379-415.
53. Lerner S, Magrane D, Friedman E. Teaching teamwork in medical education. *Mt Sinai J Med.* 2009;76:318-319.
54. Hobgood C, Sherwood G, Frush S, et al. Teamwork training with nursing and medical students: does the method matter? Results of an interinstitutional, interdisciplinary collaboration. *Qual Saf Health Care.* 2010;19:e25.
55. Weaver SJ, Dy SM, Rosen MA. Team-training in healthcare: a narrative synthesis of the literature. *BMJ Qual Saf.* 2014;23:359-372.
56. Salas E, Rosen MA. Building high reliability teams: progress and some reflections on teamwork training. *Qual Saf Health Care.* 2013;22:369-373.
57. Burke CS, Salas E, Wilson-Donnelly K, Priest H. How to turn a team of experts into an expert medical team: guidance from the aviation and military communities. *Qual Saf Health Care.* 2004;13(1):i96-i104.

9

Developing a Patient Safety Curriculum for Resident and Fellow Education

Deborah Sesok-Pizzini, MD, MBA

New Pathology Milestones From the ACGME for Patient Safety and Quality

The Accreditation Council for Graduate Medical Education (ACGME) is a nonprofit council that was established in 1981 to evaluate and accredit medical residency programs in the United States. Reform in the accreditation process happened in the late 1990s, where outcomes became the focus of residency training. The following set of six competencies became required in the 1990s by graduate medical education (GME) training programs: (1) medical knowledge, (2) communication skills, (3) professionalism, (4) patient care, (5) system-based practice, and (6) practice-based learning.[1] In the mid-2000s, concerns were raised that the current program was inadequate, and there was a push to provide more standardized training and outcomes nationally. This resulted in the redesign and implementation of the ACGME Next Accreditation System (NAS) and the Milestones project.[2-5]

Milestones in pathology were developed to evaluate resident physicians during their participation in an ACGME residency or fellowship program.[6] The intention of the milestones are for use in semiannual reviews of resident performance. Milestones are organized from less advanced to more advanced and evaluate knowledge, skills, attitudes, and other attributes. Each level of a resident's performance will be evaluated with the milestones, from level 1, where the resident is a graduate medical student experiencing the first day of residency, to level 5, where the resident has advanced beyond performance targets set for residency and is demonstrating skills that might describe someone who has several years of experience in practice. The pathology milestones are a set of descriptors that measure progress in patient care, procedural skill sets, medical knowledge, practice-based learning and improvement, interpersonal and communication skills, professionalism, and systems-based practice. Embedded in these milestones are specific outcomes and goals for patient safety and quality.

Implementation of NAS and CLER Site Visits

In the NAS, there will be fewer demands placed on residency programs, as it is intended to reduce the work to maintain accreditation for the programs in good standing. For example, programs will be assigned a 10-year interval between site visits. Pathology programs will begin the use of NAS in the spring of 2013 in phase II of the program, and the implementation of the milestones will be July 1, 2014.[7] The site visits will be a self-study using methods that are similar to those used in the Liaison Committee on Medical Education. This self-study method may include a "tracer" style that follows a patient, using a methodology similar to that used by The Joint Commission. Annual updates of the residency program will be through the web-based ACGME Accreditation Data System. Although the administrative responsibilities will be less for program directors and coordinators under NAS, the sponsoring institution (SI) will have more accountability for GME and will undergo a Clinical Learning Environment Review (CLER) site visit every 18 months.[8] The CLER site visit will focus on six issues: patient safety; quality improvement; transition of care; supervision; duty hours, fatigue management, and mitigation; and professionalism.

The SI must demonstrate to the CLER site team that it has an infrastructure to support GME by addressing five questions (see Table 9-1). During this inspection process, the CLER team will meet with the designated institutional officer (DIO), chair of the GME committee, CEO, chief medical officer, and chief nursing officer, in addition to the patient safety officer.

Table 9-1. Key Questions for a Clinical Learning Environment Review (CLER) Site Visit
What organizational structure, and administrative and clinical processes does the sponsoring institution (SI) have in place to support graduate medical education (GME) learning in the six areas?
What are the roles of GME leadership and the faculty to support learning in the above six areas?
How engaged are the residents and fellows in using the SI's current clinical learning environment infrastructure?
How does the SI determine the success of its efforts to integrate GME into the quality infrastructure?
What areas has the SI identified as opportunities for improvement?

The tracer methodology will also be used as residents escort the CLER site team on a walk-around. After meeting with all program directors, faculty members from all departments, and peer-elected housestaff, the CLER Evaluation Team Committee will prepare a report to evaluate the support for faculty and leadership development in the six areas.

Patient safety fits into ACGME accreditation with both the NAS milestones and core competencies required for CLER visits. The methods used to evaluate the milestones include (1) direct observation, (2) portfolios, (3) 360 evaluations, (4) periodic self-assessment, (5) narratives, and (6) simulations. The residents may refer to the milestones to better assess their current level of performance and future goals as they progress through residency. To assist with resident evaluations, each residency and fellowship training program must form its own clinical competency committee (CCC). The CCC consists of at least three to five faculty members representing broad disciplines in the department. The purpose of the CCC is to meet semiannually to review each resident using all possible evaluation tools and to assign the milestone level for all 29 milestones applicable. Furthermore, the CCC is an advisory board for the program director.

Examples of Advancing Through Pathology Patient Safety Milestones

When we consider patient safety milestones in pathology, we can begin with systems-based practice (SBP) 1: Patient safety: Demonstrates attitudes, knowledge, and practices that contribute to patient safety (anatomic pathology [AP] and clinical pathology [CP]). In these milestones, the most basic expectation is that the resident understands the importance of identity and integrity of the specimen, and understands the risk inherent in handoffs. Progression to level 5 requires that the resident model patient safety practices, write and implement policies on patient safety, and complete an advanced maintenance-of-certification (MOC) patient safety module. The complete milestones with levels are available on the ACGME website.[9]

The question, then, is how to promote residents from level 1 to level 5 or, at the very least, ensure that residents achieve a competency level expected when standardized nationally. Even ensuring that the goals of milestone levels 3 and 4 are reached requires the ability to teach problem-solving skills to residents so that they become more proficient in recognizing and analyzing preanalytic, analytic, and postanalytic errors. So how do you teach these skills to residents? One of the best ways is for faculty to model these skills throughout their daily work. For example, if it was necessary to deviate from a policy for good reason, was the resident available to discuss the rationale behind the decision as well as the process needed to make that decision? Was the resident able to review with you the signed deviation form? The lessons that the residents will learn from actively engaging in this process will far outweigh a lecture, which is not tied to their situational learning at the moment.

In addition to on-the-job training, where else can residents learn some of these skills? The value of simulation training is also very useful. Even if residents are not available to participate in a full root cause analysis (RCA), an RCA can be simulated in a lecture environment, where residents are each assigned to role-play one of the participants in the RCA. With some background information and some scripted dialogue, the residents quickly pick up on their character and contribution to the RCA. This can even be taken a step further by having the residents act out "good" and "bad" professionalism during an RCA. This allows the other residents who are witnessing the role-playing to comment on what can be barriers in communication based on what they observed. Other areas where simulation may be a useful tool is with education regarding handoffs, which may offer a unique learning environment to identify opportunities for improvement in a no-risk situation.[10]

The Importance of Handoffs in the Curriculum

Handoffs (or handovers) play an important role in residency training because this process is identified as a Joint Commission requirement. Because breakdowns in communication were identified as a major factor in sentinel events, The Joint Commission made handoffs a requirement as part of the National Patient Safety Goal to improve the effectiveness of communication among caregivers. The goal is to "Implement a standardized approach to handoff communications, including an opportunity to ask and respond to questions."[11-13] The process will be examined by interviewing staff to determine if they are aware of the process and if they are really doing it. Direct observation will also play a role in evaluation. Handoffs in pathology are just as important as in other areas in the hospital, such as the OR and in critical care units, and, realistically, every time a specimen changes hands is part of a handoff process. Other examples of handoffs are critical values that are reported to the ordering physician. In these situations, standardized "readbacks" may be an effective tool to improve communication accuracy.[14] Shift-to-shift handoffs occur with the laboratory staff, and incomplete laboratory work needs to be discussed, as well as critical information about testing issues and results. Residents are also involved in this handoff as information flows to them from other residents, staff, clinical caregivers outside the department, and, in some situations, like in transfusion medicine, the patients themselves.

Standardization of handoffs then become critical, and each residency program should address the best design for their institution.[15] One communication tool that is often used for handoffs is Situation, Background, Assessment, and Recommendation (SBAR).[16] This tool was developed from the military realm for the purpose of transferring concise information from one person to the other. The value of the tool is to provide a structured framework, and the tool is easily teachable to staff. Handoffs should be both written and verbal for important information, such as a critical value. Readback procedures were implemented in pathology specifically for this purpose to ensure that a test result was understood by the receiver. The topics of handoffs are addressed in more detail in chapter 4, *Communication, Handoffs, and Transitions*.

Meeting Milestones and Incorporating the Goals into Service Work, Lectures, and Real Work Experience

The Institute of Medicine (IOM) recently published their new patient safety report focusing on diagnostic error.[17] This is fundamental to the practice of pathology because as pathologists we are expected to render a diagnosis based on patient sample, either in AP or CP. For the purpose of training programs, this falls under milestones that relate to developing leadership, management, patient safety, quality improvement, and professional skills. The IOM report noted that as many as 5% of US adults who seek outpatient care each year experience a diagnostic error. In addition, postmortem examinations showed that as many as 10% of patient deaths may have resulted from a diagnostic error, and medical record reviews suggest that 6% to 17% of adverse events result from such errors. The purpose of the IOM report is to provide a broader focus to identify opportunities to improve the diagnostic process, while examining work systems and conceptual models that influence diagnostic decision making.

One of the first recommendations to improve diagnostic errors is to facilitate more effective teamwork among health care professionals, patients, and their families. This concept shows up in the interpersonal and communication skills (ICS) 1 milestone, which refers to intradepartmental interactions and development of leadership skills: Displays attitudes, knowledge, and practices that promote safe patient care through team interactions and leadership skills within the laboratory (AP/CP). An example of advancing through the milestones in this situation is to take a resident from level 1—which is characterized by demonstration of respect for and willingness to learn from all members of the pathology team—to a mastery of level 5, where the resident can lead the pathology team effectively. The residency training program should provide opportunities to enhance teamwork skills to work effectively with others as well as introduce concepts such as conflict management.[18,19] This may be taught in the settings of lectures, simulations, or case-based discussions to introduce the importance and relevance of this topic to safe patient care. In addition, active learning and experiential activities may be key in reinforcing these safety principles.[20] Exposing the resident to team activities (working in collaboration with other colleagues) will also enhance learning. This process may include multidisciplinary chart reviews, case presentations, and quality improvement initiatives that span several specialties.

Another example of milestones that address the recommendation of teamwork for safe patient care is ICS2, which addresses the importance of formulating a differential diagnosis and communicating with other team members. As a resident progresses from this level 1 milestone to level 5, the resident becomes more aware of the limitations of his or her own medical knowledge and becomes more effective as a consultant to other health care team members. The ability to discuss pathology findings with other health care members is paramount to the role of the pathologist, because these findings may have a significant impact on patient care and treatment. For example, one study showed that there is a communication gap between pathologists and surgeons. In a study where questionnaires were distributed to attending surgeons and trainees based on surgical pathology reports, results showed that surgeons misunderstood pathologists' reports as much as 30% of the time. Moreover, more experience reduced but did not eliminate this problem.[21] Therefore, providing residents with opportunities to lead multidisciplinary conferences and communicate directly with clinical colleagues about a differential diagnosis is extremely beneficial in advancing residents through the milestones to become proficient in these interactions.

A second recommendation from the new IOM report is ensuring that health information technologies support patients and health professionals in the diagnostic process. This is also addressed in the pathology milestones with specific recommendations about clinical informatics as it applies to both AP and CP. At the most basic level, a resident should demonstrate a familiarity with technical concepts of hardware, software, and operating systems. As a resident advances through training, the resident should be able to apply informatics skills as needed in a project. At a very advanced training level, the resident should participate in troubleshooting information technology issues as well as demonstrate skills to assess and purchase a laboratory information system.

Two other recent IOM recommendations are also addressed in the pathology milestones: (1) develop and deploy approaches to learn from and reduce diagnostic errors and near misses in clinical practice and (2) establish a work system and culture that supports the diagnostic process and improvements in diagnostic performance. These IOM goals are embedded in the milestone of a resident who is first functioning at level 2 for laboratory management skills, who demonstrates an understanding of when to file an incident or safety report and knows the concept of a laboratory quality management plan. A more advanced resident who is functioning at level 5 is able to utilize continuous improvement tools, such as Lean and Six Sigma, as well as manage a laboratory quality assurance and safety plan. Of interest, the IOM recommendations for a culture that supports the diagnostic process and improvements specifically refers to a nonpunitive approach to errors. This is also included in the practice-based learning and improvement (PBLI) milestone: Recognition of errors and discrepancies. Level 1 begins with acknowledging and taking responsibility for errors when recognized. This can only occur in an environment where residents feel safe disclosing and discussing errors. This type of workplace culture is best achieved by leaders who also exemplify this behavior. Residents will then reflect upon their own errors in a group setting (level 3) and progress to more advanced skills of modeling and using errors and discrepancies to improve practice (level 5).

When we discuss a nonpunitive culture in patient safety, we are often referring to the principles of a "fair and just culture" model. This framework for error analysis was first described by Marx[22] and stresses the need for caregivers to feel safe when voicing a concern. Also, this framework balances the accountability of both the individual and the organization responsible for designing the system in the workplace. This shifts the focus from errors and outcomes to system design and management of behavioral choices of all employees in an organization.[23,24] With this in mind, residents would be held accountable for a reckless decision that resulted in a patient safety event but could not be held responsible in the same way to a system design that promoted the likelihood of error. A just culture is essential for development of a high-reliability organization that promotes the continuous learning and redesigning of systems.[25]

Additional recommendations of the IOM report on diagnostic errors address a more macro system approach to developing a reporting environment and medical liability system that facilitates improved diagnosis through learning from diagnostic errors. As pathologists and pathology trainees, we can work with our societal advocacy groups to create safer environments without legal discovery to discuss diagnostic errors and near-misses. A recent article addressed the recommendations for disclosure of a medical error to patients when another clinician or trainee was involved.[26] In particular, this calls for pathologists to become part of that conversation when a laboratory error is involved.[27] If questions about test results or diagnoses arise in conversation with patients, it is better to be able to inform the patient how the error may be prevented in the future. As a specialty, we may have limited training on how to disclose an error. In fact, a recent survey showed that many pathologists feel less than satisfied with their skills in error disclosure.[28] The key to improvement will be early education and training of residents to provide them with the tools to feel more confident as an active participant in error disclosure. This will, in turn, create an improved training environment for our residents, as they learn from others' errors. In conclusion, we are encouraged to look at the payment and care delivery system and the way that this may contribute to diagnostic errors, and what we can do as a community to advocate for right action for these concerns. Lastly, funding for research on diagnostic processes and diagnostic errors will help us create future leaders in this field by introducing this area of study early on in their careers.

Giving and Receiving Resident Feedback

In many studies now, it is recognized that poor communication leads to additional safety errors. A culture that supports dysfunctional communication among caregivers is one that will have more patient safety risks. A large body of literature is now available on disruptive physician behavior and how that impacts patient safety. It is essential that trainees observe respectful communication among faculty and know that faculty are held accountable for appropriate professional, ethical, and respectful behavior.[5,29] In a training program, residents must feel comfortable to address concerns with an attending pathologist without feeling that they will be on the receiving end of an angry, impatient physician. Likewise, attending pathologists must be able to give feedback to residents about how they are progressing through their training program. All of this ties back into patient safety, as effective communication is at the core of ideal patient safety cultures. So how do you get from one place to another in building a culture of safety?

One easy solution is to model effective communication. The difficulty arises when we, as physicians, also were not trained in the best ways to communicate medical errors. Some programs have actually suggested milestones for faculty development that model the residency ACGME requirements to ensure that faculty are also meeting expectations.[30] In addition, courses are now available in "crucial conversations," which help describe a high-risk, high-emotion, and high-stakes conversation.[31] The basic premise of this coursework is to make the environment safe so that the person stays in the conversation. If the resident goes into silence (quietly passive-aggressive) or if the attending goes into violence (shouting and body language that expresses anger), problems will not be solved and potential patient safety solutions not identified. Feedback to the resident about errors that may or did impact patient safety must be given in a constructive manner.

It is best to give feedback soon after the incident occurs, while focusing on the facts and minimizing the emotional response of the persons giving and receiving feedback. This is not easy, but the more this behavior is practiced and modeled, the easier it becomes. It is recommended that you begin with "I need to give you some feedback about [the incident]" or "May I give you some feedback about…". As the attending shares the facts, it is important to listen to the resident about his or her perception of the facts. Again, the goal is to make the conversation about errors safe so that the full story of each person is understood. The value is that more information will be known and better decisions will be made in the future to address potential patient safety errors.

One potential way to model good and effective feedback is to provide video instruction in which either residents/attendings or professional actors may participate in making examples of "good" and "bad" feedback. A joint session between faculty and residents could then create the right forum for discussion of these videos and identifying areas where the communication on either side could be improved. Another way to accomplish this goal is to perform real-time simulation or role-playing on effective feedback methods. One of the challenges with this approach is that the right environment is needed so that both groups feel comfortable enough sharing and role-playing in front of each other. In our institution, we found videos to be an ideal way to present this topic. These videos can also be used for future training sessions for newer residents and faculty.

Effective feedback is an important milestone with regard to professional development. This extends past the basic level of being able to receive feedback constructively. The expectation is that the resident will not only accept the feedback, but will also modify his or her practice in response to the feedback. As residents' skills mature in feedback, they should be able to encourage and actively seek feedback as well as be able to provide constructive feedback themselves. The most skilled resident will continuously model giving and receiving constructive feedback.

Recommendations for the Advanced Resident and Resources for Teaching Patient Safety

In many residency programs, a few residents will gravitate toward the topic of patient safety and show an early passion for the literature and work that supports developing an advanced skill set in patient safety attitude, knowledge, and practices. The goal of the residency program is to create opportunities where these residents can become more advanced, reaching a level 5, and, more important, develop a passion for future work in this area. In some hospitals, councils are formed where interested residents across multiple disciplines can come together to work on hospital-wide resident quality and patient safety initiatives. An example where residents can have a significant impact is handoffs and other policies where the residents are directly involved in the work. Other training opportunities may be with professional pathology societies that offer coursework or committee work that relates to patient safety. One such example is offered by the College of American Pathologists (CAP), where residents may participate as junior members on various committees that review laboratory proficiency testing. It is important for program directors to encourage these opportunities. Other avenues may be "shadowing" a faculty member who is actively engaged in patient safety work, where the residents learn by participating in root cause analyses, failure mode effects analyses, quality improvement initiatives, and patient safety committees.

Patient Safety in Other Pathology Milestones and Continuous Patient Safety Medical Education

Patient safety is not limited to ACGME milestone SBP1. There is much overlap between patient safety and other milestones, including laboratory management, quality management, professionalism, informatics, recognition of errors and discrepancies, intradepartmental interaction and development of leadership skills, and interdepartmental and health care clinical team interactions. Therefore, developing a robust leadership and management training program along with a quality improvement curriculum will only further advance patient safety learning initiatives.[32,33] Even consultation and procedure milestones have patient safety goals embedded in them. Keeping in mind the end goal of patient safety, important factors include critical value reporting, ensuring the integrity of a specimen to avoid cross-contamination or identify mix-up, and discussion with attending staff of any requests that are contraindicated. As residents grow in their development, they appreciate, increasingly, how interconnected their work is with caring for the patient and understand that their role plays a significant part.

Every opportunity that attending pathologists use to create these conversations—as to how the task of what the resident is currently doing impacts the patient—is helpful in the training process. One way to focus on the patient is to begin each conference with a "patient safety story." These stories are vignettes that are shared at the beginning of a conference or meeting about a recent event that may or may not have impacted patient care. The value in telling the story is that others will learn and remember if they are in a similar situation next time. Also, this narrative format provides a tool to collect and analyze other unrecognized patient safety issues.[34] Other ways to promote this culture of safety is to include recognition of a "good catch."[35] When a resident or attending discovers an error and fixes it before it impacts the patient, the team celebrates by informing others through a monthly newsletter or communication on a website. One may take this a step further by actually giving an award at the end of the year for the best "good catch" or a leadership award that recognizes a resident or attending who contributed most significantly to advancing departmental goals of building a culture of patient safety.

Advanced residents are consistently able to understand the inherit risks in different processes and are very good at troubleshooting preanalytic, analytic, and postanalytic errors, as needed, without supervision. When these senior residents consistently model safety practices, they may be given additional responsibilities, including writing and implementing policies on patient safety. Because the residents are often at the "sharp end" of patient care, and many errors occur based on their actions, some training programs have suggested having a resident as a quality patient safety (QPS) officer. In an effort to engage residents in policy-making processes and to promote greater housestaff participation in quality and patient safety initiatives, one large academic medical center created a Housestaff Quality Council, appointing the Housestaff Chair of the Committee as the Resident QPS Officer.[36] The council's responsibilities include identifying QPS issues, collecting data, analyzing data, implementing process/systems changes, and monitoring the effectiveness of the changes. The creation of this type of committee and leadership will help to foster a new generation of physician leaders to further enhance the quality and patient safety goals in health care.[37]

As the resident graduates, there are opportunities to continue patient safety education using online modules provided by state or national societies. The American Board of Pathology has approved a maintenance-of-certification (MOC) program provided by the American Society for Clinical Pathology, which offers an online training course in patient safety. Other advanced training may be obtained through organizations such as the Institute for Healthcare Improvement, which sponsors a course for patient safety officers and others committed to learning more about methods and techniques to address patient safety errors and near misses. An online training module for patient safety provided by the CAP is also available and is entitled, "Creating a Culture of Patient Safety." Many journals publish papers that are related to patient safety, and lectures are offered at national societal meetings that serve as a method for continuing medical education (CME) in this field. Studies have shown that more-interactive workshops may result in changes to knowledge or skills as compared with didactic sessions alone.[38] This may help guide physicians in selecting the best opportunities for CME to transform patient safety culture at their institutions. There are also opportunities for institutional and national funding with organizations that call for research proposals with goals to advance the study and collection of data related to patient safety concerns. For example, the American Medical Association has created the National Patient Safety Foundation to sponsor research and education in the area of patient safety.[39]

Other topics related to patient safety are communicating effectively, accepting responsibility, working well in teams, leading a multidisciplinary discussion, analyzing problems, being accountable, and resolving conflicts. These concepts are not just models for patient safety practice, but also models for management and leadership. Therefore, additional training in management and leadership by pursuing coursework in a variety of venues is also beneficial in building proficiency in patient safety. It may be easier for many individuals to find training at the local level for these types of sessions because many local human resource departments at institutions sponsor these types of training seminars for their employees. Residents may either attend these sessions, or special sessions may be developed for the trainees at the different institutions modeled after the same coursework. For those wanting to pursue a more advanced education, a master of business administration or other master's or doctoral degree related to a field of management, leadership, or public health may be appropriate to advance efforts to fully engage in future patient safety activity. Some institutions are sponsoring a fellowship dedicated to "quality and patient safety," where interdisciplinary coursework is combined to create a dynamic learning environment to build on a basic structure of patient safety skills and tools. Many of these trainees will go on to become early leaders in patient safety, trained in methodology and tools to advance the field of study of health care errors and near misses.

Moving Patient Safety Metrics

The key to success of implementation of a patient safety curriculum is to ultimately develop a culture that embraces the principles of patient safety. Metrics to measure the effectiveness of a program may include surveys given to faculty and residents asking questions regarding the six areas of CLER competencies. Other metrics may include monitoring the number of monthly safety reports filed by residents and having performance targets to increase this number to encourage transparency in event reporting. Yet another metric may be direct feedback given to institutional leaders through performing patient safety walkarounds. As clinical leaders reach out to residents, faculty, and other health care providers during their daily work routine, opportunities may arise to identify best practices or areas for improvement and to develop collaborative strategies for improvement across the organization and among different training programs.

One can also assess learning via pre and post surveys or tests that are given before the resident engages in the didactic part of the curriculum and then after the training is complete. For example, programs that have focused on improving communication and handoffs may assess learning and perceptions towards personal skills in evaluation of handoffs. At one institution, after taking a pre and post survey and completing coursework that was based on nationally recognized handoff guidelines, the residents were able to more readily identify important aspects of the handoff, felt more competent in giving handoffs, and identified more clinical errors from poor handoffs.[40] This GME committee was able to show a statistically significant improvement in the area of handoffs and transitions of care, as well as in their ratings of communication and openness in "The Agency for Healthcare and Research Quality Culture of Safety Survey," given annually to both housestaff and faculty.

Curriculum for Patient Safety

As noted, patient safety education can be approached in a multitude of ways to address the basics of patient safety, which include (1) basic terminology, (2) event reporting, (3) tools for analysis, (4) systems thinking, (5) human factors and cognitive biases, and (6) a nonpunitive approach to error reporting. Many experts internal and external to the field of pathology may be available to introduce these topics to residents and fellows. It is fundamentally important that residents become engaged in the error-reporting system at their institution so that they understand the most common causes of errors and provide sharp-end feedback about how to prevent them.[41] This allows the residents to become a robust part of a highly integrated system that strives for high reliability and continuous quality improvement. An example of fundamentals and content objectives to include in a curriculum are listed in Table 9-2.

A patient safety curriculum often includes formal and informal components. A formal curriculum involves planned didactic sessions, lectures, problem-based learning, simulation, small-group teaching, quality improvement projects, and so forth. An informal or hidden curriculum is what the trainees learn each day by observing others and their relation to the work culture and system. If the residents are learning about effective communication in a formal program, but the faculty are not modeling this in the "informal curriculum," the opportunity for real culture change and improvement will be lost. Also, organizations that do not have a strong safety culture and continuous improvement mindset will struggle to have their residents engaged and interested in patient safety and quality initiatives.[42]

Other ways to promote an informal or hidden curriculum in patient safety is to formally and publicly recognize a health care team that helps reinforce patient safety principles and demonstrates best practices in this area. This team may involve physicians, nurses, pharmacists, technologists, support staff, and hospital administrators. For example, when residents receive emails from hospital administrators acknowledging their contributions for promoting patient safety, this becomes part of the informal curriculum. Other examples of an informal or hidden curriculum are discussions with residents about serious safety events, the sharing of the hospital's quality performance initiatives, and daily discussions about patient safety and quality. This is a highly experiential form of learning and is dependent on the attitudes and interactions between teacher and learner.[43]

In 2011, the World Health Organization *Multiprofessional Patient Safety Curriculum Guide* was developed to ensure that patient safety education is delivered in an integrated way. The guide is divided into two parts: part A provides the background for educators on how to select and teach each topic and integrate the topics into the institution's current curriculum; part B describes 11 patient safety topics that

Developing a Patient Safety Curriculum for Resident and Fellow Education

Table 9-2. Core Curriculum for Patient Safety Resident Education

Topic	Content Objectives
Introduction to importance of patient safety and the Institute of Medicine report	Understand the reason that patient safety is so critical to patient care and resident education
Introduction to event reporting	Institutional mechanism to report, detect, and review errors
Introduction to error types in pathology	Preanalytic, analytic, and postanalytic errors
Introduction to patient safety classification	Joint Commission–based performance, near-miss and actual serious safety events
Introduction to how errors are made	Reason's Swiss cheese model, knowledge, rule-based performance, skill-based performance
Introduction to cognitive bias	Fast and slow thinking, analytical deductive reasoning (slow), using rules, pattern-recognition (fast)
Causes and contributory factors	Human factors and system failures (organizational and technical), including information technology, which both contributes to and prevents error
Introduction to event analysis	Flow charts, failure mode and effects analysis, root cause analysis, apparent cause analysis, fishbone diagrams
Teaching teamwork, communication, professionalism	Giving and receiving feedback, handoffs, effective communication, raising concerns to leaders, disruptive physicians, conflict management, leadership, managing self and others, coaching employees, emotional intelligence, building relationships
Safety behaviors for error prevention	Introduction, Situation, Background, Assessment, Recommendation, make time for Questions/Answers (ISBARQ); cross-checking and coaching; readback; paying attention to detail; supporting each other; mindfulness
Continual review of safety events	Resident meetings, participation in root cause analysis, discussion and review of recent safety reports, telling of safety stories, patient safety simulations
Disclosing medical error	Risk management, communicating medical errors, accountability, patient relations, patient stories
Fair and just culture and response to patient adverse events	Nonpunitive approach to errors; identifying negligence, recklessness, intentional rule violations; supporting the caregiver; second victim; system failures
Quality improvement	Quality tools, quality performance measurements, statistical process improvements, data management and reporting, run charts, quality initiatives, participation in quality improvement projects
Changing and evolving culture	Building awareness and accountability, organizational learning, physicians leading patient safety and quality improvement efforts, proactive risk mitigation, high-reliability organization, modeling behavior

Learning activities may include lectures, case-based discussions, small-group sessions, departmental and interdepartmental patient safety and quality conferences, resident engagement in patient safety and quality initiatives and projects, simulations, video vignettes, leadership modeling, journal clubs, online institutional or national society training, and national conferences.

cover a range of core material[44] (see Table 9-3). The value of this curriculum guide is that it is designed to be used across specialties, and it is intended to take patient safety beyond the classroom. This curriculum includes health professional "buddying," role-modeling, hospital-based improvement and team-based learning projects, independent studies, and simulation training. It also provides a link to websites and other resources for learners and educators.

James Reason once said in an interview that his famous "Swiss cheese model" for system errors was developed while making tea and feeding his cat. He noted the number of slips that one could make when they were not mindful during that process[45] (see Figure 9-1). If there were not proper defenses in place, it was easy to see how each mistake could continue forward, resulting in an ultimate accident or error. In a time where young trainees have so much data available to them,

Table 9-3. World Health Organization (WHO) Patient Safety Curriculum Topics

What is patient safety?
Why applying human factors is important for patient safety
Understanding systems and the effect of complexity on patient care
Being an effective team player
Learning from errors to prevent harm
Understanding and managing clinical harm
Using quality improvement methods to improve care
Engaging with patients and care givers
Infection prevention and control
Patient safety and invasive procedures
Improving medication safety

From WHO *Multi-professional Patient Safety Curriculum Guide*.[44]

with the expectation of assimilating this data quickly and correctly for a diagnosis, it is important to teach the concepts of slowing down when needed in order to complete a task, communicate a handoff, or coach a fellow resident on a proper technique. In the future, the agenda for patient safety will involve the power of multidisciplinary teams, reaping the benefits of information technology, supporting national and international agendas for patient safety, and putting our patients first.[46] It is our responsibility to encourage the residents to identify latent errors that are embedded in the system design of workflow and procedures that increase opportunities for failures and patient safety risks. Ultimately, our goal is not only to improve the residents' ability to detect and recover from errors, but also to train the next generation of pathologists to be the change agents for the system to promote safer patient care.

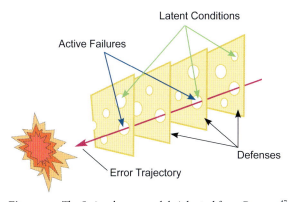

Figure 9-1. The Swiss cheese model. Adapted from Reason.[47]

References

1. Swing SR. The ACGME outcome project: retrospective and prospective. *Medical Teacher.* 2007;29: 648-654.
2. Nasca TJ, Philibert I, Brigham T, Flynn TC. The next GME accreditation system: rationale and benefits. *N Eng J Med.* 2012;366(11):1051-1056.
3. Weiss KB, Wagner R, Nasca TJ. Development, testing, and implementation of the ACGME clinical learning environment review (CLER) program. *J Grad Med Educ.* 2012;4(3):396-398.
4. Weiss KB, Bagian JP, Wagner R, Nasca TJ. Introducing the CLER Pathways to Excellence: a new way of viewing clinical learning environments. *J Grad Med Educ.* 2014;6(3):608-609.
5. Deitte L. The new residency curriculum: professionalism, patient safety, and more. *J Am Coll Radiol.* 2013;10:613-617.
6. The Pathology Milestone Project. *J Grad Med Educ.* 2014;6(1 Suppl 1):182-203.
7. Naritoku WY, Alexander CB, Bennett BD, et al. The pathology milestones and the next accreditation system. *Arch Pathol Lab Med.* 2014;138:307-315.
8. Clinical Learning Environment Review (CLER) program. Accreditation Council for Graduate Medical Education. http://www.acgme-nas.org/cler.html. Accessed October 2, 2015.
9. Pathology ACGME Milestones. Accreditation Council for Graduate Medical Education. https://www.acgme.org/acgmeweb/tabid/142/ProgramandInstitutionalAccreditation/Hospital-BasedSpecialties/Pathology.aspx. Accessed March 11, 2016.
10. Pukenas EW, Dodson G, Deal ER, Gratz I, Allen E, Burden AR. Simulation-based education with deliberate practice may improve intraoperative handoff skills: a pilot study. *J Clin Anest.* 2014;26:530-538.
11. National Patient Safety Goals 2007. The Joint Commission. http://www.jointcommission.org/PatientSafety/NationalPatientSafetyGoals/07_npsgs.htm. Accessed October 2, 2015.
12. JCAHO's 2006 National Patient Safety Goals: handoffs are biggest challenge. *Hosp Peer Rev.* 2005;30(7): 89-93.
13. Croteau R. JCAHO comments on handoff requirement. *OR Manager.* 2005;21(8):8.
14. Prabhakar H, Cooper JB, Sabel A, Weckbach S, Mehler PS, Stahel PF. Introducing standardized "readbacks" to improve patient safety in surgery: a prospective survey in 92 providers at a public safety-net hospital. *BMC Surg.* 2012;12:8.
15. Starmer AJ, Spector ND, Srivastava R, et al. Changes in medical errors after implementation of a handoff program. *N Engl J Med.* 2014;371(19):1803-1812.
16. Pope BB, Rodzen L, Spross G. Raising the SBAR: how better communication improves patient outcomes. *Nursing.* 2008;38(3):41-43.
17. Balogh EP, Miller BT, Ball JR, eds. *Improving Diagnosis in Health Care.* Washington, DC: National Academies Press; 2015.

18. Weller J, Boyd M, Cumin D. Teams, tribes and patient safety: overcoming barriers to effective teamwork in healthcare. *Postgrad Med J.* 2014;90:149-154.
19. Brandler TC, Laser J, Williamson AK, Louie J, Esposito MJ. Team-based learning in a pathology residency training program. *Am J Clin Pathol.* 2014;142: 23-28.
20. Singh R, Naughton B, Taylor JS, et al. A comprehensive collaborative patient safety residency curriculum to address the ACGME core competencies. *Med Educ.* 2005;39:1195-1204.
21. Powsner SM, Costa J, Homer RJ. *Arch Pathol Lab Med.* 2000;124:1041-1046.
22. Marx, D. *Patient Safety and the "Just Culture": A Primer for Health Care Executives.* New York, NY: Trustees of Columbia University in the City of New York; 2001.
23. Boysen PG II. Just culture: a foundation for balanced accountability and patient safety. *Ochsner J.* 2013;13:400-406.
24. Yates GR, Bernd DL, Sayles SM, Stockmeier CA, Burke G, Merti G. Building and sustaining a system-wide culture of safety. *Jt Comm J Qual Patient Saf.* 2005;31(12):684-689.
25. Johnson JK, Miller SH, Horowitz SD. Systems-based practice: improving the safety and quality of patient care by recognizing and improving the systems in which we work. In: Heriksen K, Battles JB, Keyes MA, Grady ML, eds. *Advances in Patient Safety: New Directions and Alternative Approaches. Vol. 2: Culture and Redesign.* Rockville, MD: Agency for Healthcare Research and Quality; 2008.
26. Gallagher TH, Mellow MM, Levinson W, et al. Talking with patients about other clinicians' errors. *N Engl J Med.* 2013;369(18):1752-1757.
27. Cohen DA and Allen TC. Pathologists and medical error disclosure: don't wait for an invitation. *Arch Pathol Lab Med.* 2015;139:163-164.
28. Dintzis SM, Stetsenko GY, Sitlani CM, Gronowski AM, Astion ML, Gallagher TH. Communicating pathology and laboratory errors: anatomic pathologists' and laboratory medical directors' attitudes and experiences. *Am J Clin Pathol.* 2011;135:760-765.
29. Speck RM, Foster JJ, Mulhern VA, Burke SV, Sullivan PG, Fleisher LA. Development of a professionalism committee approach to address unprofessional medical staff behavior at an academic medical center. *Jt Comm J Qual Patient Saf.* 2014;40(4):161-167.
30. Shag D, Goettler CE, Torrent DJ. Milestones: the road to faculty development. *J Surg Educ.* 2015;72(6):226-235.
31. Patterson K, Grenny J, McMillan R, Switzler A, eds. *Crucial Conversations: Tools for Talking When Stakes Are High.* New York, NY: McGraw-Hill; 2012.
32. Hemmer PR, Karon BS, Hernandez JS, Cuthbert C, Fidler ME, Tazelaar HD. Leadership and management training for residents and fellows. *Arch Pathol Lab Med.* 2007;131:610-614.
33. Boonyasai RT, Windish DM, Chakraborti C, Feldman LS, Rubin HR, Bass EB. Effectiveness of teaching quality improvement to clinicians. *JAMA.* 2007;298(9):1023-1037.
34. Cox LM, Logio LS. Patient safety stories: a project utilizing narratives in resident training. *Acad Med.* 2011;86(11):1472-1478.
35. Herzer KR, Mirrer M, Xie Y, et al. Patient safety reporting systems: sustained quality improvement using a multidisciplinary team and "good catch" awards. *Jt Comm J Qual Patient Saf.* 2012;38(8):339-347.
36. Fleischut PM, Evans AS, Nugent WC, Faggiani SL, Kerr GE, Lazar EJ. Call to action: it is time for academic institutions to appoint a resident quality and patient safety officer. *Acad Med.* 2011;86(7):826-828.
37. Leotsakos A, Ardolino A, Cheung R, Zheng H, Barraclough B, Walton M. Educating future leaders in patient safety. *J Multidiscip Healthc.* 2014;7:381-388.
38. Mazmanian PE, Davis DA. Continuing medical education and the physician as a learner: guide to the evidence. *JAMA.* 2002;288(9):1057-1060.
39. Classen DC, Kilbridge PM. The roles and responsibility of physicians to improve patient safety within health care delivery systems. *Acad Med.* 2002;77(10):947-952.
40. Allen S, Caton C, Cluver J, Mainous AG III, Clyburn B. Targeting improvements in patient safety at a large academic center: an institutional handoff curriculum for graduate medical education. *Acad Med.* 2014;89(10):1366-1399.
41. Samulski TD, Montone K, LiVolsi V, Patel K, Baloch Z. Patient safety curriculum for anatomic pathology trainees: recommendations based on institutional experience. *Adv Anat Pathol.* 2016;23(2):112-117.
42. Myers JS, Nash DB. Graduate medical education's new focus on resident engagement in quality and safety: will it transform the culture of teaching hospitals? *Acad Med.* 2014;89:1328-1330.
43. Singh R, Naughton B, Taylor JS, et al. A comprehensive collaborative patient safety residency curriculum to address the ACGME core competencies. *Med Educ.* 2005;39:1195-1204.
44. WHO Patient Safety Curriculum Guide. World Health Organization. http://www.who.int/patientsafety/education/curriculum/en/. Accessed March 29, 2017.
45. Peltomaa K. James Reason: patient safety, human error, and Swiss cheese. *Q Manage Health Care.* 2012;21(1):59-63.
46. Hilborne LH, Lubin IM, Scheuner MT. The beginning of the second decade of the era of patient safety: implications and roles for the clinical laboratory and laboratory professionals. *Clin Chim Acta.* 2009;404:24-27.
47. Reason J. Human error: models and management. *BMJ.* 2000;320:768-770.

10

Patient Safety and the Patient Navigator

Elizabeth A. Wagar, MD

Introduction:
What Is a Patient Navigator?

The traditional management of patient care in the United States is self-directed by the patient or through the efforts of family members or designated family sponsors, either legally defined through so-called *living wills* or informally, as recognized by individual state legal systems. After 1950, as insurance benefits began to be provided as an employee benefit, more complicated payment systems evolved, including complex coverage agreements. The coverage agreements extended to physician selection, by the use of physician networks and practice groups. New payment mechanisms included deductible amounts—that needed to be met before coverage ensued—and copay arrangements. Complexity was added at the physician level by the development of federal coding mechanisms for medical necessity (International Classification of Diseases, Revision 10 [ICD-10]) and procedure-based payments using Current Procedural Terminology (CPT) codes.

The complexity of health care also increased exponentially and simultaneously, making it difficult for individuals and patients' families to "navigate" the health care system. *Patient navigators* evolved as consultants who assist patients in the management of their health care in a given health care system. The occupation originally developed from the perspective of the insurance industry. As such, they evaluate insurance options and resolve insurance and billing disputes. They may, for example, handle appeals of claims and negotiate access to specific clinical services or medication in the insurance arena. Under federal health care law, federal and state-sponsored health insurance exchanges must hire navigators to help individuals and businesses evaluate and enroll in supplemental health care plans. For Medicare patients selecting pharmaceutical coverage under Medicare Part D, for example, individual enrollees interact with a patient navigator who assists in choosing a plan that gives best value and best coverage on the basis of their current health care conditions. As such, patient navigators, until recently, were primarily employees of insurance companies or contractors or employees of agencies assisting in Medicare enrollment.

The concept of a patient navigator has expanded to include handling of more-complex health care scenarios and, as such, has sometimes merged with the term *patient advocate*. Patient-centric advocacy appeared during the patient's rights movement of the 1970s. Probably the first advocacy organization in the United States was the National Welfare Rights Organization (NWRO). The NWRO was developed in the 1960s by Lillian Craig, from Cleveland, Ohio, who fought for the rights of individuals reliant upon government welfare. It brought attention to welfare programs and emphasized their value. It also enhanced the funding of welfare programs but ceased to exist in the mid-1970s.[1]

The NWRO was the original source of The Joint Commission accreditation standards related to patients' rights. The NWRO preamble eventually became the basis for the Patients' Bill of Rights, which was acknowledged by the American Hospital Association in 1972.[2,3] The Patients' Bill of Rights is now prominently posted in all Joint Commission-accredited hospitals in the United States. The most frequent themes identified in a given institution's patients' bill of rights are shown in Table 10-1. Health advocacy and patient advocacy have different goals. Health advocacy tends to work for the larger good, from a public health care perspective. An example of an organization focused on the larger good is the American Cancer Society. In contrast, what has developed at the patient-centric level is the field of patient advocacy and patient navigators.

The perception of the role of patient navigator as a professional occupation is a relatively recent development. A profession organizes around three elements: association, credentialing, and education. Established in 1980, the Master's Program in Health Advocacy at Sarah Lawrence College was probably the first formal educational effort toward defining the profession.[2] The Society for Healthcare Consumer Advocacy became an association that principally represented hospital-based patient advocates. It is a member association of the American Hospital Association. As employers, however, hospitals exerted employer rights and have, in some respects, left the roles of patient navigators and patient advocates somewhat in limbo at the professional level. Patient advocacy and patient navigation still remain somewhat distinct but may overlap in services, depending on the employer and the health care organization.

Table 10-1. Frequency of American Hospital Association Patients' Bill of Rights Themes in State Statutes and Hospital Documents

Theme The patient has a right to:	State Statutes (= 23), %	Hospital Documents (= 240), %
Considerate and respectful care	78	97
Obtain current and understandable information	87	93
Refuse recommended treatment	87	97
Have an advanced directive	35	95
Privacy	87	93
Confidential communications and records	78	92
Review records	43	88
Indicated medical care including transfer to another facility	39	90
Be informed of business relationships that influence care	17	40
Refuse participation in research	74	58
Reasonable continuity of care	43	87
Be informed of charges as well as policies for patient responsibilities and resolution of conflicts	74	57

From Paasche-Orlow MK et al.[35] Reproduced with permission of Springer.

In 2006, patient advocates assembled in Shelter Rock, Long Island, New York, to discuss the need for a professional association of patient-centric health advocates. After several meetings of patient advocates, the summation was the development of the National Association of Healthcare Advocacy Consultants. The organization does not have specific educational or credentialing requirements. It holds annual meetings of patient-centric professionals who are defined as patient advocates or patient navigators by their employment. However, it extends the reach of the profession, offering resource connections for training, development of competencies, and professionalism; it also has a code of ethics that all members must agree to when joining the organization.[4]

Present-Day Patient Navigator/ Patient Advocacy Roles

The complexity of health care has increased, especially as clinical care became more specialized and technology more advanced. Oncology is probably the first specialty to use the patient navigator or patient advocate professional for comprehensive health care management. Examining the route of patient care in a primary diagnosis of breast cancer exemplifies this complexity (Figure 10-1). As many as six physicians may be required for patient care in this scenario, with the patient visiting a similar number of specialty clinics, depending on the organization of the health care providers.

What is the role of a patient navigator or patient advocate? The definition of health care advocacy excludes direct, hands-on care, which is a clear distinction between advocacy and patient diagnosis and treatment. Given these exclusions, the patient navigator or advocate can perform multiple functions: (1) financial consultation for evaluation of coverage/insurance options, (2) facilitation of the appointment process, (3) conversations that clarify care so that the patient is able to make informed clinical decisions, (4) supportive referrals for related long-term care and chemotherapy side effects, and (5) supportive referrals for family and caregivers.

Financial consultation provides clarification of the patient's insurance coverage. This is one of the original functions of the patient navigator and still exists as a single type of navigation support for federal programs such as Medicare. Through this process, the patient navigator can assist a patient in making best choices, dealing with deductible amounts, clarifying maximums such as annual and lifetime maximum coverages, and coverage of pharmaceuticals. A patient dealing with a crisis can be in need of this logical and well-informed support while managing his or her personal care.

Facilitation of the appointment process is more likely to be a function of a given institution's patient navigator or advocacy support. Some institutions with linked care for oncology, surgery, and radiology can assure proper timing of appointments through the physician's office. This may not always be the case, however, in complex care situations. A patient advocate can review an appointment schedule with the patient and assist with any gaps or rescheduling. Large cancer centers frequently have a patient advocacy

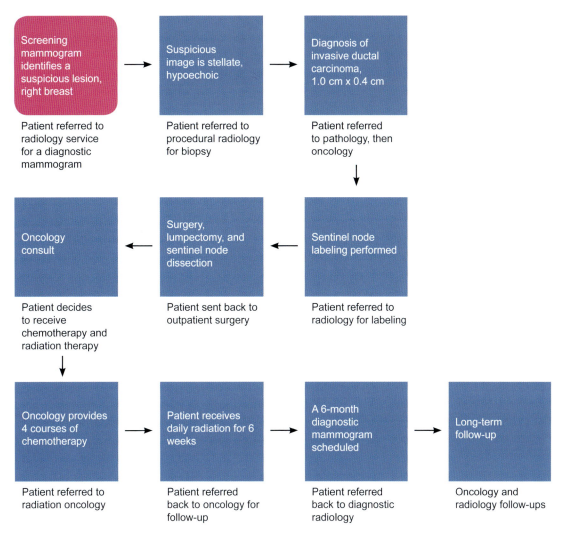

Figure 10-1. Process diagram of time to diagnosis and time to treatment for a diagnosis of primary breast cancer.

office that assists in the coordination of the appointment process.

It is ultimately the physician's responsibility to make clear the selection of treatment options; however, with the advent of electronic informational resources, patients may be confused, and a patient advocate can assist in clarifying the questions or identifying areas of misunderstanding. Often the physician has limited appointment time for discussion. The patient advocate can spend the time required to further clarify options; however, the patient advocate or navigator must avoid making recommendations and incomplete profiling of the health care situation faced by a patient in the midst of a major health care scenario.

A patient navigator can also assist with secondary follow-up issues such as chemotherapy side effects. Typically the oncologist will refer for significant side effects, such as cardiac failure. However, the patient navigator can assist the patient in understanding all possible side effects so that the patient can pursue appropriate referrals with his or her physician. Also, psychological and psychiatric consultations may be available. Services may range from group therapy sessions for cancer patients to monthly "grand rounds" for cancer patients, presented at the lay level. A patient advocate can assist in identifying the availability of such services.

Finally, a patient advocate or navigator can assist family members and caregivers. The consultations for family members may include available rehabilitation services, hospice services, and psychological support for the spouse and for children. A navigator can help a caregiver find a variety of other services that simply support family needs, from food delivery to break periods for caregivers. In addition, the assessment of needs for legal services has been recommended as consistent with the emerging trends of patient-centric treatment.[5]

Implementation of Patient Navigator/Advocate Systems

Most formal patient navigator/advocate systems have been implemented through the efforts of funded research, typically in oncology, as a means for addressing disparities in socioeconomic factors and timely cancer care. In the early 1990s, Harold Freeman aimed to reduce delays in care for disadvantaged populations by addressing barriers to care through one-on-one interventions.[6] Systems have expanded rapidly so that by 2003, more than 200 navigation programs were reported.[7] Other national efforts include the American Cancer Society, the Centers for Medicare and Medicaid Services' Medicare Cancer Prevention and Treatment Demonstration for Racial and Ethnic Minorities, and the National Cancer Institute Patient Navigation Research Program.[8-11]

The Boston Cancer Institute Patient Navigation Research Program reported results that indicated navigation produced more timely resolution after abnormal screening.[10] However, the variability in such programs is considerable, involving the level of navigator training, the portfolio of services provided, the outcomes measurement, and the efficacy. The lack of reimbursement also significantly inhibits the development of programs. The variability in services provided and the lack of standardization still limit most measurements and ultimately most assumptions regarding outcomes. It should be noted, however, that the Commission on Cancer mandated that all accredited cancer centers implement patient navigation programs by 2015. With this accreditation action, more comparative evaluations may soon become available.

The Evidence for Improved Patient Care

As previously mentioned, Dr. Freeman at Harlem Hospital in New York City developed the first formal patient navigator system.[12] He observed that the economically disadvantaged encountered significant barriers to cancer care and often lacked relevant information to make decisions regarding their diagnoses. In his early survey, the combination of free or low-cost examinations with navigation yielded a significantly higher percentage of early-stage disease and a greater number of patients surviving 5 years (from 39% to 70%).[13] As we examine the evidence, however, we must remember that Dr. Freeman's patient population was one that encountered significant barriers to clinical care.

Most of the recent literature regarding patient navigators/advocates has focused on breast cancer and/or colorectal cancer diagnosis and treatment management. A study by Basu et al[14] examined the timely diagnosis of patients with breast cancer, using a nurse navigator program. Because navigation services are required for accreditation by the National Accreditation Program for Breast Centers, these services are becoming more prevalent nationally. During two 9-month intervals, breast cancer patients diagnosed with stage 0 to II were identified by retrospective review. Overall, 176 patients met the inclusion criteria: 100 before and 76 after nurse navigation implementation. Nurse navigation was found to significantly shorten the time to consultation for patients older than 60 years. This was a short-term analysis but seemed to indicate a quality improvement in time to diagnosis for older patients.[14]

Battaglia et al[10] performed a controlled study to assess the impact of patient navigation in a population defined as vulnerable based on federal funding for inner-city community health care centers as the selected sites for study. The study included women who had either breast or cervical abnormal screening tests; 997 women were examined during baseline, and 3041 women were examined during navigation regarding time to diagnosis, adjusting for covariates, clustering by clinic and difference from baseline. For cervical abnormalities, there was a significant decrease in time to diagnosis in the navigated group and among those with a breast cancer screening abnormality that resolved after 60 days, with no difference before 60 days. The conclusion was that time to diagnosis can be improved in patients identified as belonging to a lower income group.[10]

A study by Hoffman et al[15] reviewed the effects of navigation versus nonnavigation on 2601 patients: 1047 navigated patients were compared with 1554 nonnavigated patients receiving diagnoses of breast cancer. In this study, the diagnostic time (days) was significantly shorter for navigated patients (25.1 days) as compared with nonnavigated women (42.1 days). Subanalysis indicated that patients in which biopsies were performed, in particular, reached diagnostic resolution faster in the navigated patient group.[16]

In contrast, a study by Fiscella et al[16] showed no overall benefit using intent-to-treat analysis for patients receiving diagnoses of breast or colorectal cancer. The study compared randomized groups to baseline for a total of 438 patients. Patients were randomized to two groups, one with patient navigators and one without. No statistically significant difference was noted in time to completion of primary cancer treatment. Subgroup analysis showed higher satisfaction in socially disadvantaged patients. The findings also point out the difficulties in measuring some outcomes data such as psychological distress. Their results also emphasize the original proposition of Dr.

Freeman that the socially disadvantaged seem to reap the most benefits. Also, another mixed cancer study by Wells et al,[17] combining breast and colorectal cancer screening, showed little impact on the overall time to completion of diagnostic care (1267 total patients: 588 navigated and 679 controls). Although more navigated patients achieved diagnostic resolution by 180 days, the results were not statistically significant. The strength of the studies by Battaglia[10] and Hoffman,[16] however, still suggest that time to treat is an important variable to consider.

A study in Tampa, Florida, examined 1039 patients reviewed for abnormal breast cancer screening results (494 navigated patients, 545 controls). In this study, the adjusted hazard ratio was examined and the results suggested that navigation had no effect on resolution time in the first 3 months. However, navigated patients reached diagnostic resolution more quickly when compared with the control group at longer intervals; at 4.7 months, a reduced time to diagnosis was noted.[18]

Several studies that have specifically examined navigated intervention for colonoscopy and colorectal cancer screening show varying results depending on study objectives. Lee et al[19] looked at the cost effectiveness of navigation intervention and expectedly showed an increased cost per participant for navigated patients. The Moffitt Patient Navigator Research Program examined a small group of patients (75 navigated and 118 controls). The adjusted time-varying navigator effect on diagnostic resolution was marginally significant, with a lagged effect at more than 4 months, and the adjusted hazard ratio showed a lagged effect at 12 months.[19] The longer time resolution seems to be a pattern, but it must be noted that different cancer grades and stages are incorporated into many of these studies. Also, the income disparities are not consistently evaluated.

A colorectal cancer screening was evaluated in a rural setting and compared low-income patients (n = 809) at multiple clinics. Those patients who attended navigated clinics were significantly more likely than patients at comparison clinics to undergo colonoscopy and be guideline compliant on screening tests. Again, the lower income socioeconomic group seems to show best improvement when patient navigation is implemented.[20]

Some of the most recent studies have focused on hospitalizations and rehospitalizations, which are a recognized negative health outcome; this metric has legitimacy also as a federal metric for quality of health care in the United States. A study by Balaban et al[21] examined in-network, 30-day hospital readmissions stratified by patient age and with recognized readmission risk factors. There were 585 intervention patients and 925 controls. Overall, 30-day readmission rates for the patients older than 60 years showed a significant decrease of 4.1% in readmission.[21] From the cancer perspective, survivorship and hospital admission are important markers of quality outcomes. In a study at the University of Alabama, patients were followed both before and after navigation implementation in the University of Alabama Health System Cancer Community Network (19,335 beneficiaries). Patients were older than 65 years with a diagnosis of cancer and were followed for 2 years. The study was able to show significant decreases in hospitalizations, emergency room visits, and intensive care unit admissions, and an increase in hospice use. There was a pre/post decrease in health care costs of $952 per beneficiary.[22]

In summary, patient navigation/advocacy is in the very early stages of implementation. Several studies have shown value to the patient by decreasing the time to diagnostic resolution and decreasing hospital admissions and readmissions. Most of the studies have been performed in cancer screening and diagnosis scenarios, and the types of personnel serving as navigators or advocates vary in educational level and background. In addition, many of the studies are nonspecific with respect to tumor type and grade, complicating the variety of outcomes, especially given recent advances in specialized molecular tumor typing. There is a general sense, however, in reviewing the literature, that patient navigators or advocates shorten the time to diagnosis in cancer, especially for patients who are socioeconomically disadvantaged. Also, it appears that decreasing hospital admissions and readmissions may be an important effect for patient navigation and advocacy.

The Patient Navigator/Advocate and Patient Safety

Patient safety is the prevention of adverse effects to patients, avoiding errors, and learning from the errors that do occur. Patient safety became a highly public issue when the report from the Institute of Medicine, *To Err Is Human,* was published in 2000.[23] This publication was quickly followed by another from the Institute of Medicine, *Crossing the Quality Chasm.*[24] Wide publicity ensued, and the culture of the health care systems became a focus of the discussion. Safety, as described by Cook,[25] is a characteristic of systems and not their components, and is an emergent property of systems. Health care is one of the most complex systems that individuals (patients) interface with in the course of a lifetime. Patient navigation and advocacy is an interesting development in the field of patient safety, given that the purpose of the navigation and advocacy model is to assist patients with the *system* of health care. Thus, navigation and advocacy may play a valuable role in the course of developing safe mechanisms for all aspects of the health care interface.

To date, the actual proof that navigation and advocacy contribute to patient safety is somewhat limited. The two examples discussed here are time to diagnosis and hospitalization/rehospitalization. In the field of oncology, the timeliness of initiation of adjuvant chemotherapy has long been examined. A meta-analysis focusing on the trials of perioperative chemotherapy for breast cancer showed an apparent benefit to its early initiation, with a reduced risk of relapse of 11%.[26] Retrospective analyses have produced more conflicting results[27-29]; however, retrospective analysis has some weaknesses related to arbitrary cutoff points and a full understanding of the grade and stage of the disease. Current guidelines provided by the European Society of Medical Oncology on the timing of adjuvant chemotherapy for breast cancer indicate that treatment should start preferably within 2 to 6 weeks of diagnosis. A significant decrease in the efficacy of chemotherapy is observed when administered more than 12 weeks after surgery.[30] This finding may generate future studies investigating the interventions of patient navigation.

More recently, the biology of specific breast cancer tumor types has been acknowledged as a factor in the timing of adjuvant chemotherapy. For example, in a study by Gagliato et al[31] of 6827 patients, no differences were seen between cohorts starting chemotherapy at 0 to 30 days versus 31 to 60 days, or more than 60 days after surgery. However, when viewed from the perspective of stage, patients with more-advanced-stage disease had worse outcomes if chemotherapy started more than 60 days after surgery. Also, patients with triple-negative breast disease and those with HER2-positive tumor treated with trastuzumab had a worse overall survival if chemotherapy was started more than 60 days after surgery.[31] Obviously, the biology and heterogeneity of the various tumor presentations plays a role and indeed makes the recommendation process for the timing of chemotherapy treatment complex. It is unlikely at this time that a survey using a randomized, controlled trial for timing of adjuvant chemotherapy will occur, considering the problems related to recruitment and ethics. Despite the controversial evidence, it is suspected that it may be unwise to unnecessarily delay the initiation of adjuvant chemotherapy in patients for whom the impact of such therapy is expected to be significant.[32] This finding may represent another opportunity for patient navigators.

The earlier-described data by Battaglia[10] and Hoffman[15] suggest that the intervals of time to diagnosis and time to treat can be decreased by the use of patient navigation/advocacy.[10,15] Although other studies also suggest variability in these results, one of the positive aspects of a patient navigation/advocacy program appears to be more efficient delivery of patients to subsequent surgery and chemotherapy for breast cancer.[10,15,33] For some subpopulations, for example older patients, this effect was more pronounced. These findings suggest that patient navigation/advocacy may well be one of the mechanisms by which patient safety can be improved in terms of patient outcomes and long-term survival. Further research is obviously required. However, it makes sense that a program that covers the health care system as a whole, rather than its components, should be a valuable tool in improving patient safety.

Another area where patient navigation/advocacy may play an important role is in hospitalization/rehospitalization of patients, particularly those with chronic conditions. In the Affordable Care Act, a Hospital Readmissions Reduction Program requires the Centers for Medicare and Medicaid Services to reduce payments to hospitals with excess readmission.[34] Readmission measures for acute myocardial infarction, heart failure, and pneumonia were to be established, with expansion to chronic obstructive pulmonary disease, total hip arthroplasty, and total knee arthroplasty in 2015. The study by Balaban et al[21] clearly shows that with patient navigator intervention, readmissions were decreased for patients older than 60 years, with a statistically significant adjusted decrease of 4.1%. These data suggest that patient navigator/advocacy programs can affect patient safety by reduced readmissions in the elderly. Perhaps this is not surprising, given that such programs reflect the system of health care as compared with its individual components.

An exciting aspect of patient navigation/advocacy is the investigations that have not yet been developed regarding patient safety. As a systems-based program, the use of a patient navigator or patient advocate can help prevent misunderstood appointment times, as an example. A knowledgeable advocate may be able to check for laboratory results, ascertain the ordering sequence of procedures within an algorithm, and provide advice to patients regarding medication compliance. The variety of patient safety investigations that can be considered expands dramatically once a full understanding of the relationship of patient safety to the continuum of patient care is appreciated. Patient safety and patient navigation/advocacy are natural partners for the future investigation of major patient safety initiatives.

References

1. National Welfare Rights Organization. Ohio History Central www.ohiohistorycentral.org/w/National_Welfare_Rights_Organization?rec=1663. Accessed November 10, 2016.
2. Master of Arts in Health Advocacy at Sarah Lawrence College. www.sarahlawrence.edu/health-advocacy. Accessed November 10, 2016.
3. Rothman, D. *Beginnings Count*. New York: Oxford Press; 1997.
4. Code of Ethics. National Association of Healthcare Advocacy Consultants. www.nahac.com/code/. Accessed September 15, 2016.
5. Retkin R, Antoniadis D, Pepitone DF, Duval D. Legal services: a necessary component of patient navigation. *Semin Oncol Nurs*. 2013;20:149-155.
6. Freeman H, Muth B, Kerner J. Expanding access to cancer screening and clinical follow-up among the medically underserved. *Cancer Pract*. 1995;3:19-30.
7. Hede K. Agencies look to patient navigators to reduce cancer care disparities. *J Nat Cancer Inst*. 2006;98:157-159.
8. Gunn C M, Clark JA, Battaglia TA, Freund KM, Parker VA. An assessment of patient navigator activities in breast cancer patient navigation programs using a nine-principle framework. *Health Serv Res*. 2014;49:1555-1577.
9. Mitchell JB, Haber SG, Holden DJ, Hoover S. *Evaluation of the Cancer Prevention and Treatment Demonstration for Ethnic and Racial Minorities: Second Report to Congress*. Research Triangle Park, NC: RTI International; 2010.
10. Battaglia T, Bak S, Heeren T, et al. Boston Patient Navigation Research Program: the impact of navigation on time to diagnostic resolution after abnormal cancer screening. *Cancer Epidemiol Biomark Prev*. 2012;21:1645-1654.
11. Esparza A. Patient navigation and the American Cancer Society. *Semin Oncol Nurs*. 2013;29:91-96.
12. Freeman HP. Cancer in the socioeconomically disadvantaged. *CA Cancer J Clin*. 1989;39:266-288.
13. Oluwole SF, Ali AO, Ad A, et al. Impact of cancer screening programs on breast cancer stage at diagnosis in a medically underserved urban community. *J Am Coll Surg*. 2003;196:180-188.
14. Basu M, Linebarger J, Gabram SGA, Patterson SG, Amin M, Ward KC. The effect of nurse navigation on timeliness of breast cancer care at an academic comprehensive cancer center. *Cancer*. 2013;119:2524-2531.
15. Hoffman H J, LaVerda NL, Young HA, et al. Patient navigation significantly reduces delays in breast cancer diagnosis in the District of Columbia. *Cancer Epidemiol Biomark Prev*. 2012;21:1655-1663.
16. Fiscella K, Whiteley E, Hendren S, et al. Patient navigation for breast and colorectal cancer treatment: a randomized trial. *Cancer Epidemiol Biomark Prev*. 2012;21:1673-1681.
17. Wells K J, Lee J-H, Calcano ER, et al. A cluster randomized trial evaluating the efficacy of patient navigation in improving quality of diagnostic care for patients with breast or colorectal cancer abnormalities. *Cancer Epidemiol Biomark Prev*. 2012;21:1664-1672.
18. Lee J-H, Fulp W, Wells KJ, Meade CD, Calcano E, Roetzheim R. Patient navigation and time to diagnostic resolution: results for a cluster randomized trial evaluating the efficacy of patient navigation among patients with breast cancer screening abnormalities, Tampa, FL. *PLOS One*. 2013;8:e74542.
19. Lee J-H, Fulp W, Wells KJ, Meande CD, Calcano E, Roetzheim R. Effect of patient navigation on time to diagnostic resolution among patients with colorectal cancer-related abnormalities. *J Cancer Educ*. 2014;29:144-150.
20. Honeycutt S, Green R, Ballard D, et al. Evaluation of a patient navigation program to promote colorectal cancer screening in rural Georgia, USA. *Cancer*. 2013;119:3059-3066.
21. Balaban R B, Galbraith AA, Burns ME, Vialle-Valentin CE, Larochelle MR, Ross-Degnan D. A patient navigator intervention to reduce hospital readmissions among high-risk safety-net patients: a randomized controlled trial. *J Gen Intern Med*. 2015;30:907-915.
22. Rocque GB, Pisu M, Jackson BE, et al. Trends in resource utilization and costs during implementation of a lay navigation program [abstract]. *J Clin Oncol*. 2015;33(Suppl):Abstract 6502.
23. Kohn LT, Corrigan JM, Donaldson MS, eds; Committee on Quality of Health Care in America; Institute of Medicine. *To Err is Human: Building a Safer Health System*. Washington, DC: National Academy Press; 2000.
24. Richardson WC, Berwick DM, Bisgard JC, eds; Committee on Quality of Health Care in America; Institute of Medicine. *Crossing the Quality Chasm: A New Health System for the 21st Century*. Washington, DC: National Academy Press; 2001.
25. Cook, RI. Two years before the mast: learning how to learn about patient safety. In: Hendee WR, ed. *Enhancing Patient Safety and Reducing Errors in Health Care*. Chicago, IL: National Patient Safety Foundation; 1998.
26. Clahsen PC, Van de Velde CJH, Goldhirsch A, et al. Overview of randomized perioperative polychemotherapy trials in women with early stage breast cancer. *J Clin Oncol*. 1997;15:2525-2535.
27. Shannon C, Ashley S, Smith IE. Does timing of adjuvant chemotherapy for early breast cancer influence survival? *J Clin Oncol*. 2003;21:3792-3797.
28. Cold S, During M, Ewerta M, et al. Does timing of adjuvant chemotherapy influence the prognosis after early breast cancer? *Br J Cancer*. 2005;93:627-632.
29. Lehrisch C, Paltiel C, Gelmon K, et al. Impact on survival of time from definitive surgery to initiation of adjuvant chemotherapy for early-stage breast cancer. *J Clin Oncol*. 2006;24:4888-4894.
30. Senkus E, Kyriakides S, Penault-Llorca F, et al. Primary breast cancer: ESMO Clinical Practice Guidelines for diagnosis, treatment and follow-up. *Ann Oncol*. 2013;24(Suppl 6):vi7-32.

31. Gagliato DDM, Gonzalez-Angulo AM, Lei X, et al. Clinical impact of delaying initiation of adjuvant chemotherapy in patients with breast cancer. *J Clin Oncol.* 2014;32:735-744.
32. Colleoni M, Gelver RD. Time to initiation of adjuvant chemotherapy for early breast cancer and outcome: the earlier, the better? *J Clin Oncol.* 2014;22:717-719.
33. Freund KM, Battaglia TA, Calhoun E, et al; for the Writing Group of the Patient Navigation Research Program. Impact of patient navigation on timely cancer care: the Patient Navigation Research Program. *J Nat Cancer Inst.* 2014;106(6):dju115.
34. Readmissions Reduction Program (HRRP). Centers for Medicare and Medicaid Services. https://www.cms.gov/Medicare/Medicare-Fee-for-Service-Payment/AcuteInpatientPPS/Readmissions-Reduction-Program.html. Updated April 18, 2016. Accessed September 15, 2016.
35. Paasche-Orlow MK, Jacob DM, Hochhauser M, Parker RM. National survey of patients' bill of rights statutes. *J Gen Intern Med.* 2009;24(4):489-494.

Index

Accreditation Association for Ambulatory Health Care (AAAHC), 3
Accreditation Council for Graduate Medical Education (ACGME), 33-35, 101-102
    Accreditation Data System, 101
    Clinical Learning Environment Review (CLER), 101-102, 107
    Milestones project, 101-104
    Next Accreditation System (NAS), 101
Agency for Healthcare Research and Quality (AHRQ), 3
    20 Tips to Help Prevent Medical Errors, 3
American Association of Blood Banks (AABB), 67
American Medical Association, 39
American Society for Clinical Pathology (ASCP), 1, 106
Association of Directors of Anatomic and Surgical Pathology (ADASP), 30, 31
    recommendations for critical diagnoses, 30, 31
Automation, role of, in the laboratory, 22-23
Autoverification, 22, 50

Barcoding, 8, 12, 23, 43, 46, 48-49
    in anatomic pathology, 56
    in point-of-care testing (POCT), 55
    in transfusion medicine, 56

Centers for Disease Control and Prevention (CDC), 3, 5
Centers for Medicare and Medicaid Services (CMS), 10, 11, 114, 116
Clinical and Laboratory Standards Institute (CLSI), 13, 67, 68
Clinical Laboratory Improvement Amendments of 1988 (CLIA '88), 10, 19, 20, 30, 67, 69
Clinical Learning Environment Review (CLER), 101-102
Cognition, pathologist, 75-78
Cognitive abilities and associated skills, 72
Cognitive bias and diagnostic errors, 71-85
    examples of cognitive biases, 82-83
Cognitive errors, examples in anatomic and clinical pathology, 75
Cognitive failures, 73
Cognitive heuristics, 79-80
College of American Pathologists (CAP), 1, 61, 105
    Creating a Culture of Patient Safety, 106
    Laboratory Accreditation Program (LAP), 30
    Q-Probes, 12, 13, 29, 68
    Q-Tracks, 13, 29, 68
    recommendations for dealing with critical diagnoses, 30, 31
Common cause variation, 61
Communication, 104-105, 108
    barriers to effective, 96
    between resident and attending, 32
    of final surgical, cytologic, or autopsy diagnosis, 33
    importance of, 29-30
    requirements for effective, 37-38
    tools for effective, 38-39
Communication, handoffs, and transitions, 29-41
Computerized provider order entry (CPOE), 43-48, 56, 69
    clinical decision support (CDS), 46
    collection instructions, 47
    corollary orders, 45
    CPOE order sets, 45
    CPOE search and screen modifications, 45-46
    and electronic health record (EHR), 46
    implementation, 46
    ordering messages and alerts, 44-45
    order provider identification, 47
    responsible provider, 53
    and specimen collection systems, 46-47
    specimen processing, 47
Control charting, 61-62
Crew resource management (CRM), 25, 96
Critical values reporting, 30-31, 51, 52
    automated reporting systems, 53
    flagging abnormal/critical results, 52
Culture of patient safety, 4, 5-18
Curriculum for resident and fellow education, 101-110
    ACGME Milestones project, 101-104
    ACGME Next Accreditation System (NAS), 101
    Clinical Learning Environment Review (CLER), 101-102, 107
    core curriculum for patient safety resident education, 107-108
    importance of handoffs in, 102-103
    metrics to measure effectiveness of, 107
    resident feedback, giving and receiving, 104-105
    Swiss cheese model, 108-109
    WHO *Multi-professional Patient Safety Curriculum Guide*, 107-108, 109

DMAIC (defining, measuring, analyzing, improving, checking), 64, 65

Eindhoven classification model, 73
Electronic health record (EHR), 46, 68-69
    abnormal/critical results, 52-53
    clinical decision support (CDS), 46
    CPOE implementation, 46
    external result entry, 55
    interfaces to, 51
    and point-of-care testing (POCT) results, 55
    and reference laboratory testing, 55
    SAFER Guides, 69
    specimen collection systems, 46-47
    test result review, 51-52
    tests pending at discharge, 53-54

Index

Error analysis, 63-67
Error collection, 63
Error reporting and follow-up, 13-14
Errors, 73
    Joint Commission classification of causes of, 74
Errors, diagnostic, 1, 80-82
    and cognitive bias, 71-85
Errors, frequency of, 1-2
Errors, in anatomic pathology, 12
    monitoring, 12-13
Errors, in clinical pathology
    analytic, 8-9
    monitoring, 12-13
    in point-of-care testing (POCT), 10-11
    postanalytic, 9-10
    preanalytic, 6-8
Errors, laboratory, defined by cause, 6
Errors, medical, management of, 1
Evaluating patient safety in the laboratory, 61-70
Event-reporting systems, 63

Failure mode and effects analysis (FMEA), 22-23, 61, 65-66, 67, 105, 108
Flow charts, 61
Food and Drug Administration (FDA), 8, 10, 11, 67
Fordism, 71
Framing, 35

Getting the board on board, 97-98

Handoffs, 31, 71
    approach to the standardization and measurement of, 35
    between primary clinicians, 34
    in graduate medical education, 33-34
    importance of, in resident and fellow education, 102-103
    in pathology graduate medical education, 36-37
    in resident and fellow education, 102-103, 105, 107, 108
    Targeted Solutions Tool (TST), 38
Hand-overs, 31, 97, 102. *See also* Handoffs
Health information technology (HIT), 68-69
High-reliability organizations (HROs), 87-90
    definition, 88-89
    organization design, 89-90
High-reliability teams, 91-94
    structure, 92-93
Human Factors Analysis and Classification System (HFACS), 67, 73
Human factors and ergonomics (HFE), 19-22, 25, 26
    SEIPS (Systems Engineering Initiative for Patient Safety) model, 20
    work system components, 20-22
Human factors and patient safety, 19-27

Infobuttons, 51, 54
Institute for Healthcare Improvement (IHI), 63, 64, 97, 106
Institute for Medical Quality, 3
Institute of Medicine (IOM), 1, 2, 3, 29, 61, 68, 103-104
    Crossing the Quality Chasm: A New Health System for the 21st Century, 19, 29, 88, 115

Improving Diagnosis in Health Care, 1, 2, 29
To Err is Human: Building a Safer Health System, 1, 2, 19, 29, 71, 87, 88, 115
Instrumentation, 47
Instrument interfaces, 49
ISBAR/ISBARQ (Identify, Situation, Background, Assessment, Recommendation, Questions), 39, 97

Joint Commission, The, 3, 13, 102
    classification of causes of error, 74
    National Patient Safety Goals, 3, 30
    Patient Safety Event Taxonomy, 73, 74
    requirement for record and readback process, 37-38
    SHARE, 38-39
Joint Commission Center for Transforming Healthcare, 31, 38
    Targeted Solutions Tool (TST), 38
Just culture, 4, 14, 26

Laboratory information system (LIS), 48
    abnormal/critical results, 52-53
    autoverification, 22, 50
    LIS Functionality Assessment Toolkit, 69
    manual results entry, 49
    middleware, 51
    and point-of-care testing (POCT) results, 55
    and quality assurance, 49
    and reference laboratory testing, 55
    results interpretation, 54
    specimen collection systems, 46-47
Lapse errors, 56
Lean management, 63-64, 71
Lean thinking, 20
Levey-Jennings chart, 61-62

Mistakes, 73
Modular automation, 22

National Academy of Medicine (NAM), 19. *See also* Institute of Medicine (IOM)
National Patient Safety Foundation, 3
National Patient Safety Goals, 3, 30
National Quality Forum (NQF), Never Events, 3
National Welfare Rights Organization (NWRO), 111

Organization design, 89-90

PACT (Priority, Admissions, Changes, and Tasks), 35
Pareto chart, 65-66
Patient navigator, 111-118
    and improved patient care, 114-115
    Patients' Bill of Rights, 111, 112
    role in hospitalization/rehospitalization of patients, 115, 116
    roles, 112-113
    systems, implementation of, 114
Patient safety, definition, 5
Patient safety culture
    evolution of, 2-3
    just culture, 4, 14, 26
Patient Safety Event Taxonomy, 73, 74

Index

Patient Safety Improvement Corp, 3
Patient safety initiatives, 3-4
Patients' Bill of Rights, 111, 112
Pattern recognition, 73, 75
    cognitive strategies in, 79-80
Plan, do, check, act, 64-65
Point-of-care testing (POCT), 10-11
    and technology interfaces, 55

Q-Probes, 12, 13, 29, 68
Q-Tracks, 13, 29, 68
Quality assurance, 29
Quality control, 29
Quality improvement, 2-3
Quality System Essentials (QSEs), 67-68

Radio-frequency identification (RFID), 48-49, 57
Readbacks, 37-38
Risk priority number (RPN), 66
Root cause analysis (RCA), 66-67, 102

SAFER Guides, 69
Safety I, 71-72, 83
Safety II, 71, 72, 83-84
Safety science, 71-72
Sign-offs, 31. *See also* Handoffs
Situation, Background, Assessment, and Recommendation (SBAR), 103
Six Sigma, 64
Slips, 73
Spaghetti diagram, 24
Special cause variation, 61
Specimen collection
    instructions, 47
    systems, 46-47
Specimen processing, 47
Specimen tracking. *See also* Barcoding
    radio-frequency identification (RFID), 48-49, 57
    specimen identification and barcoding, 48-49
Statistical process control, 61-62
    control/run charting, 61-62
    flow charts, 61
Surveillance systems, 63
Swiss cheese model, 108-109
Systems Engineering Initiative for Patient Safety (SEIPS) model, 20
Systems thinking, 20, 90

Targeted Solutions Tool (TST), 38
Team building and managing, 93-94
Teams, fatigue, stress, and scheduling, 25-26
    crew resource management (CRM), 25, 96
Teamwork, 90-92
    barriers to, 96
    benefits of, 91
    critical characteristics of, 91-92
    stages of, 94-96
    teaching, 98
    using, to effect change, 96-97
Technology, system, and process issues, 23-24

Technology in laboratory patient safety, 43-60
    in analytic phase, 47-51
    anatomic pathology specimen tracking, 57
    automation, role of, in the laboratory, 22-23
    autoverification, 22, 50
    collection instructions, 47
    computerized provider order entry (CPOE), 43-47, 69
    corollary orders, 45
    CPOE implementation, 46
    CPOE order sets, 45
    CPOE search and screen modifications, 45-46
    critical values reporting, 30-31, 51, 52, 53
    electronic health record (EHR), 46, 51-55, 68-69
    external result entry, 55
    flagging abnormal/critical results, 52-53
    health information technology (HIT), 68-69
    infobuttons, 51, 54
    instrumentation, 47
    instrument interfaces, 49
    interfaces to electronic health record, 51
    laboratory information system (LIS), 22, 46, 47, 48, 50, 51, 52-53, 55, 69
    LIS and quality assurance, 49
    manual results entry, 49
    metrics and analytics, 55-56
    middleware, 48, 51
    ordering messages and alerts, 44-45
    order provider identification, 47
    point-of-care testing (POCT) results, 55
    in postanalytic phase, 51-55
    in preanalytic phase, 43-47
    radio-frequency identification (RFID), 48-49, 57
    reference laboratory testing, 54
    reflex testing protocols, 51
    responsible provider systems, 53
    result interpretation, 54
    result review, 49-50
    specimen collection systems, 46-47
    specimen identification and barcoding, 48-49
    specimen processing, 47
    test selection, 43
    tests pending at discharge, 53-54
    transfusion medicine, 56
Test selection, 43
Tests pending at discharge, 53-54
Total automation, 22
Total Quality Management (TQM), 20, 71
Total testing process, 62-63
Toyota Production System (TPS), 20, 63, 64, 71
Transfusion medicine, 22-23, 56
Transgender patients, 9, 10
Transitions, patient care, 31-33

Variation, 61
Violations, 73

Westgard rules, 8, 62, 75
Work system, components of, 20-22
World Health Organization (WHO), 5, 31
    Patient Safety Curriculum Guide, 107-108, 109

121

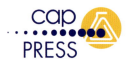